Group Treatment
for
Sexually Abused Children

JOAN GOLDEN MANDELL
LINDA DAMON

with

PAUL C. CASTALDO, EVA S. TAUBER
LAURETTA MONISE, NACHAMA F. LARSEN

Illustrations by Susan Hall-Marley

A Project of the San Fernando Valley Child Guidance Clinic

THE GUILFORD PRESS
New York   London

© 1989 The Guilford Press
A Division of Guilford Publications, Inc.
72 Spring Street, New York, NY 10012

Printed in the United States of America

This book is printed on acid-free paper.

Last digit is print number: 9 8 7 6 5

Library of Congress Cataloging-in-Publication Data

Group treatment of sexually abused children/ Joan Golden Mandell and Linda Damon with Paul C. Castaldo . . . [et al.]; illustrations by Susan Hall-Marley.
    p.   cm.
"A product of the San Fernando Valley Child Guidance Clinic."
    Bibliography: p.
    Includes index.
    ISBN 0-89862-516-5
    1. Child molesting—Handbooks, manuals, etc. 2. Sexually abused children—Rehabilitation—Handbooks, manuals, etc. 3. Group psychotherapy for youth—Handbooks, manuals, etc. 4. Child molesters—Rehabilitation—Handbooks, manuals, etc. I. Mandell, Joan Golden. II. Damon, Linda. III. Castaldo, Paul C. IV. San Fernando Valley Child Guidance Clinic.
RJ506.C48G76 1989
618.92'8583—dc20   89-7462
                                                               CIP

About the Authors

Joan Golden Mandell, MSW, LCSW, Coordinator, Family Crisis Service, San Fernando Valley Child Guidance Clinic, Northridge, California.

Linda Damon, PhD, Director of Child Abuse Services, San Fernando Valley Child Guidance Clinic, Northridge, California.

Paul C. Castaldo, MSW, LCSW, clinical social worker, Santa Clarita Valley Special Children's Center, Santa Clarita, California; former member of Family Crisis Service professional staff.

Eva S. Tauber, MSW, LCSW, Coordinator of Sexual Abuse Services, Santa Clarita Valley Special Children's Center, Santa Clarita, California; former member of Family Crisis Service professional staff.

Lauretta Monise, MSW, LCSW, clinical social worker, Family Crisis Service, San Fernando Valley Child Guidance Clinic, Northridge, California.

Nachama F. Larsen, MA, MFCC, staff therapist, Family Crisis Service, San Fernando Valley Child Guidance Clinic, Northridge, California.

The illustrator, Susan Hall-Marley, PhD, is a staff psychologist with the Family Stress Program, San Fernando Valley Child Guidance Clinic, Van Nuys, California.

98018

Acknowledgments

The authors would first like to thank all of the students and volunteers who served as cotherapists, enabling us to plan, evaluate, and refine this treatment program. Second, we are grateful for the invaluable feedback from the children and their caretakers, which taught us about the profound influence of sexual molestation on emotional development. Third, we acknowledge the support of the Robert Ellis Simon Foundation for this project by providing the funding to produce the curriculum. Fourth, an expression of appreciation goes to Susan Hall-Marley, whose illustrations enriched the presentation of the exercises. Finally, we would like to extend a special thanks to Lee Mandell, whose skill with the computer greatly facilitated the preparation of this manual.

Contents

Introduction   1

     Effects of Sexual Abuse on Latency-Age Children   1
     The Value of Group Treatment   2
     The Treatment Curriculum   3
     About This Manual   4
     References   5

CHAPTER ONE   Selection and Preparation for Group Participation   7

     Selection of Children for Group   7
     Selection of Caretakers for Group   8
     Preparation of Children for Group   10
     Preparation of Caretakers for Group   11
     Summary   13
     Caretaker Contract for Group Treatment   15

CHAPTER TWO   General Guidelines for Structure and Format of the Groups   17

     The Children's Groups   18
     The Caretakers' Parallel Groups   20
     Preparation for Group   21

CHAPTER THREE   The Curriculum   23

MODULE 1   Welcome to Your Group   27

MODULE 2   Making Friends   43

MODULE 3   Feelings Are OK   59

MODULE 4   Telling Each Other What Happened   75

MODULE 5   Telling the Secret   95

MODULE 6   My Family   113

MODULE 7   Taking Care of Myself   129

MODULE 8   Growing Up for Girls   143

MODULE 9   Growing Up for Boys   151

MODULE 10   Saying Good-Bye   159

Introduction

The San Fernando Valley Child Guidance Clinic has been providing mental health services to children and families since 1962. In 1983, the Clinic received funding from the State of California to develop and administer a specialized program (named the Family Crisis Service) to offer evaluation and treatment to identified or suspected victims of sexual abuse (ages 7–13) and their families. The professional staff determined that in order to provide effective therapeutic services, intervention must consider the impact of sexual molestation and disclosure on the children's capacity to accomplish the critical developmental tasks during the stage of latency.

EFFECTS OF SEXUAL ABUSE ON LATENCY-AGE CHILDREN

Sexual abuse can influence the acquisition of latency skills in a number of significant ways. In incest families, the sexual overstimulation can produce a chronic pattern of inappropriate sexualized behaviors, leading to prostitution or perpetration by the victims. Second, the nonoffending parent often has difficulty setting limits or rules (especially after disclosure of the abuse), which can result in confusion for a child whose sense of boundaries has been disrupted, eliciting severe testing of limits.

In cases of extrafamilial as well as intrafamilial molestation, the child who maintains silence is often preoccupied with intrusive thoughts and fears, leaving little energy for concentration in school. The victim may also experience sleep disturbances, and the resulting fatigue interferes with learning. Inability to work productively in school can lead to feelings of helplessness and inadequacy rather than competence and achievement. In addition, depression and psychosomatic symptoms, along with self-destructive and suicidal gestures, are common sequelae for molested children. Later on, substance abuse frequently occurs in adolescents and adults attempting to dull their emotional pain.

There are also several ways in which the experience of sexual abuse interferes with the development of mutually satisfying relationships with peers. Because these children have been betrayed and exploited by trusted adults, they create a barrier that interferes with their ability to establish trusting relationships. In addition, these children are often discouraged from forming relationships outside the family unit, and there is little opportunity to practice appropriate social skills. Furthermore, these children invariably experience severe guilt and shame, which reinforces their isolation and impedes their capacity for friendships. These victims are often pseudomature, and as they assume more adult role responsibilities, the gap widens even further between their peers and themselves.

Many victims of sexual abuse have not experienced adequate boundaries and therefore do not respect the rights of others. The need to defend against the intense feelings of vulnerability may translate into aggressive or sexual exploitation of others as a defense against helplessness and in an effort to achieve a sense of control. For male victims, this attempt at mastery may be even more pervasive when the debilitating effects of stigmatization and overwhelming feelings of shame lead to a profound need to reassert masculinity. Diminished self-esteem may lead to either distancing or defensive provocative behavior to alienate others further.

Eventually, the normal physiological changes that occur during late latency and early adolescence produce increased doubt and confusion in these children, who worry that they may have been damaged by the molestation. Girls may believe that menstruation is really a direct result of having been torn or cut during penetration, and they are often preoccupied with worries about whether they are still considered to be "virgins." Severe sexual anxiety and guilt can interfere with later sexual development.

Boys and their parents, on the other hand, are often consumed with anxiety that the homosexual nature of their sexual experience has somehow resulted from their inherent weakness. There is often much confusion about sexual identity, with strong fears that the boys are now or will become homosexual. In addition, parents may believe that their sons will become perpetrators, and may communicate that anxiety to their sons. Therefore, the entire process of puberty is often anticipated with significant uncertainty and dread.

Finally, the duration, extent, and frequency of the molestation, the nature of the relationship between the perpetrator and the victim, and the use of force and threats to prevent disclosure are all relevant factors that mediate the impact of the abuse on these children (Browne & Finkelhor, 1986). For further discussion of the effects of sexual molestation, the authors suggest Sgroi (1982), Gelinas (1983), and Rogers and Terry (1984). Additional information on the special issues of latency-age children can be found in Bornstein (1951), Harter (1977, 1983), Lewis (1971), Powell (1979), Sarnoff (1976, 1987), and Solnit, Call, and Feinstein (1979).

THE VALUE OF GROUP TREATMENT

Considering the important tasks of latency and the ways in which sexual abuse interferes with a child's progress through this phase, therapy must not only help the child recover from the numerous traumatic effects of sexual molestation; intervention must also be geared to the enhancement of age-appropriate skills. The benefits of group psychotherapy and the effectiveness of a structured format for child victims have been well documented in the literature (Colman, Coffey, & Myers, 1985; Damon & Waterman, 1986; Golden & Romans, 1983; Haugaard & Reppucci, 1988; Knittle & Tuana, 1980; Sturkie, 1983).

The group therapy process focuses on improved socialization by encouraging healthy interaction with peers and teaching children to respect themselves and the rights of others through maintaining appropriate boundaries. The function of group psychotherapy at this age is primarily to aid in organizing drives into socially acceptable behaviors (Kraft, 1979). The group also serves to strengthen impulse control and reality testing, and to improve self-esteem. This modality can provide latency-age victims with the reassurance that others of like age have similar scary and confusing feelings, which can be explored in a safe, supportive, and validating environment. Therefore, group treatment is often the treatment of choice for sexual abuse victims, because it decreases isolation, promotes improved social interaction, and provides the ideal setting where the children can begin to address the various conflicts surrounding the molestation. However, it is often extremely difficult for these children to talk spontaneously about the abuse experience and its aftermath, and they become easily bored, restless, and distracted without adequate structure. A nondirective approach may also collude with the secrecy that is often a dynamic in these children.

THE TREATMENT CURRICULUM

Based on the experience of treating and supervising many groups of sexually abused victims, the authors have determined that a structured and directive group treatment program can assist latency-age children to experience relief, achieve confidence and mastery, develop age-appropriate defenses, and enjoy the beginnings of mutually respectful and gratifying friendships. In addition, the inclusion of parallel treatment groups for caretakers offers nonoffending parents and guardians the opportunity to examine their own feelings and concerns about the sexual molestation, thereby increasing their capacity to understand the effects of this trauma on the development and functioning of the victims.

To achieve these goals, the issues and conflicts must be addressed in a nonthreatening manner through a systematic and long-term group treatment program. A comprehensive curriculum allows the children and caretakers to explore the sequelae of sexual molestation and to integrate extremely complicated and conflicted feelings. Moreover, the children are in a developmental phase in which discomfort and conflict are often manifested in behavioral symptoms rather than in more direct verbal communication. In order for therapy to be useful for them, material must be introduced in a way that will decrease anxiety and allow the children to guard newly acquired defenses. A program in which themes are organized and presented in a sequence of progressive difficulty, and in which these themes coincide with comfort and confidence in the group setting, significantly enhances the treatment experience for both children and caretakers. In addition, a long-term program allows children the opportunity to *work through* the feelings and conflicts in a safe, supportive setting over a significant period of time.

Finally, the prevalence of corresponding concerns and reactions of the children and the adults is an important variable in the treatment. For example, when the caretakers exhibit a strong objection to a particular group activity, the children often display a similar resistance. The authors have developed a great respect for the power of the parallel process, and believe that integration of parallel caretaker–child issues is critical to the success of the treatment for the children.

In summary, the development of a comprehensive, developmentally focused treatment curriculum:

1. Provides a structure that reinforces an awareness and respect for boundaries, decreases anxiety, and gives clear direction to the children, their caretakers, and the therapists.
2. Clarifies the therapists' expectations of the group.
3. Insures that all of the salient issues of the molestation and disclosure within the context of the latency period will be emphasized in a formal way and given appropriate significance.
4. Allows for material to be arranged and introduced in a sequence that corresponds to the children's and the adults' readiness.
5. Provides formalized activities that help children to organize their thoughts, thereby increasing their sense of mastery.
6. Lends itself well to research endeavors and decreases the time needed to prepare less experienced therapists.
7. And, finally, provides direction for the concurrent caretakers' groups.

ABOUT THIS MANUAL

On the pages that follow, the authors present a treatment curriculum for sexually abused children and their caretakers which is a compilation of experiences, ideas, and guidelines to use in the preparation and facilitation of a parallel group treatment program. It is hoped that the information in this manual will help to create interest in the challenge of providing group treatment for this population and will bolster the confidence of the experienced as well as the beginning psychotherapist.

This manual describes a sequence of treatment modules containing a variety of specific activities designed to engage the children and the adults in the group process. In addition to an explanation of how to use each activity, common resistances to the material and complementary or alternative interventions are discussed. While the program has been designed for use with both sexes, the authors recognize that there are gender differences in the response to sexual molestation and its aftermath. Where appropriate, activities and interventions that directly address the special concerns of female or male victims are explained.

It is hoped that the reader will find this structured program to be a useful tool in treatment planning. However, the authors do caution that this curriculum should serve primarily as a guideline and is not a substitute for sound clinical judgment and skill. In addition, modifications may be required, depending upon the needs of a particular community and staffing pattern. When it is more feasible to offer short-term or open-ended group programs, the selection and order of the activities can be adjusted. Finally, although this manual is designed for group treatment with latency-age children, it can also serve as a guide for individual work and many of the exercises can be used with adolescents. The same progression of modules can be used to systematically address issues in individual or family treatment, deleting those activities that can only be introduced in a group format.

The material in this manual is arranged in the following order:

CHAPTER 1. *Selection and Preparation for Group Participation*
In this chapter, the authors present important criteria for evaluating children and caretakers for inclusion in group. The chapter also discusses preparation of families for the group experience and addresses common concerns of both children and adults prior to entering group treatment.

CHAPTER 2. *General Guidelines for Structure and Format of the Groups*
This chapter provides general considerations for planning and conducting the children's and the caretakers' groups and includes the goals for parallel group treatment.

CHAPTER 3. *The Curriculum*
This chapter describes the organization of the treatment curriculum, which consists of 10 modules with specific goals and a choice of activities that can be selected to fit the needs of a particular group.

The modules are then presented in the following order:

1. WELCOME TO YOUR GROUP
2. MAKING FRIENDS
3. FEELINGS ARE OK
4. TELLING EACH OTHER WHAT HAPPENED
5. TELLING THE SECRET
6. MY FAMILY
7. TAKING CARE OF MYSELF
8. GROWING UP FOR GIRLS
9. GROWING UP FOR BOYS
10. SAYING GOOD-BYE

REFERENCES

Bornstein, B. (1951). On latency. *Psychoanalytic Study of the Child, 6*, 279–285.

Browne, A., & Finkelhor, D. (1986). Impact of child sexual abuse: A review of research. *Psychological Bulletin, 99*, 66–77.

Colman, R., Coffey, L., & Myers, P. (1985, August). *Treatment of sexual abuse with children/ adolescents in residential facilities.* Paper presented at the annual meeting of the American Psychological Association, Los Angeles.

Damon, L., & Waterman, J. (1986). Parallel group treatment of children and their mothers. In K. MacFarlane et al., *Sexual abuse of young children* (pp. 244–298). New York: Guilford Press.

Gelinas, D. (1983). The persisting negative effects of incest. *Psychiatry, 46*, 312–332.

Golden, J., & Romans, L. (1983, April). *Group treatment of sexually abused adolescent girls and their mothers.* Paper presented at the annual meeting of the American Orthopsychiatric Association, Boston.

Harter, S. (1977). A cognitive-developmental approach to children's expression of conflicting feelings and a technique to facilitate such expression in play therapy. *Journal of Consulting and Clinical Psychology, 45*(3), 417–432.

Harter, S. (1983). Cognitive-developmental considerations in the conduct of play therapy. In C. E. Schaefer & K. J. O'Connor (Eds.), *Handbook of play therapy* (pp. 100–125). New York: Wiley.

Haugaard, J. J., & Reppucci, N. D. (1988). *The sexual abuse of children* (pp. 261–292). San Francisco: Jossey-Bass.

Knittle, B. J., & Tuana, S. J. (1980). Group therapy as primary treatment for adolescent victims of intrafamilial sexual abuse. *Clinical Social Work Journal, 8*(4), 236–242.

Kraft, I. A. (1979). Group therapy. In S. I. Harrison (Ed.), *Basic handbook of child psychiatry* (Vol. 3, pp. 159–180). New York: Basic Books.

Lewis, M. (1971). *The elementary school age child. Clinical aspects of child development* (pp. 119–145). Philadelphia: Lea & Febiger.

Powell, G. J. (1979). Psychosocial development: Eight to ten years. In J. D. Call, J. D. Noshpitz, R. L. Cohen, & I. N. Berlin (Eds.), *Basic handbook of child psychiatry*, (Vol. 1, pp. 190–203). New York: Basic Books.

Rogers, C. M., & Terry, T. (1984). Clinical intervention with boy victims of sexual abuse. In I. R. Stuart & J. G. Greer (Eds.), *Victims of sexual aggression: Treatment of children, women and men* (pp. 105–124). New York: Van Nostrand Reinhold.

Sarnoff, C. A. (1976). *Latency.* North Vale, NJ: Jason Aronson.

Sarnoff, C. A. (1987). *Psychotherapeutic Strategies in the Latency Years.* North Vale, NJ: Jason Aronson.

Sgroi, S. (1982). *Handbook of clinical intervention in child sexual abuse.* Lexington, MA: Lexington Books.

Solnit, A. J., Call, J. D., & Feinstein, C. B. (1979). Psychosexual development: Five to ten years. In J. D. Call, J. D. Noshpitz, R. L. Cohen, & I. N. Berlin (Eds.), *Basic handbook of child psychiatry* (Vol. 1, pp. 186–190). New York: Basic Books.

Sturkie, K. (1983). Structured group treatment for sexually abused children. *Health and Social Work*, 229–308.

CHAPTER ONE | Selection and Preparation for Group Participation

Children and caretakers must be carefully screened and prepared prior to joining a therapy group, in order to maximize the possibility of a successful experience for all group members. In determining the appropriateness of group treatment, therapists should consider both individual (e.g., the developmental level of the child and degree of symptomatology) and situational (e.g., family dysfunction and parental psychopathology) variables. Decisions can only be made on a case-by-case basis, following a thorough psychosocial assessment. This chapter describes specific issues and guidelines in the selection and preparation phases that will help therapists to make informed choices about inclusion and facilitate each family's adjustment to the group process.

SELECTION OF CHILDREN FOR GROUP

Pragmatically speaking, careful screening of potential group members in an agency practice is often an unaffordable luxury. However, therapists should strive to complete a formal clinical evaluation with every family being considered for the group treatment program. Sufficient time must be devoted to gathering enough information to understand presenting symptomatology (including posttraumatic reactions) in the context of early developmental history, premorbid personality, and past and present family experiences and dynamics. In addition, careful assessment of ego functioning and of the quality of interactions with siblings and peers will enable therapists to make an informed determination about suitability for this program.

When evaluating a family's capacity to benefit from the structured group approach, therapists must consider whether the child possesses an adequate level of social and emotional skills:

1. The child must be able to respond to limit setting, and display adequate control of impulses with assurance that he/she does not pose a severe threat to others' safety. (Children with a diagnosis of Attention Deficit Disorder may not be able to function within the context of a contained group environment. Even with medication, these children often become too

restless and distracted, inadvertently disrupting the group. However, ADD children should not be ruled out on the basis of diagnosis alone, but evaluated for inclusion on a case by case basis.) In addition to observing the child during individual and family interviews, it is most advisable to confer with school personnel for more extensive feedback on how well the potential group candidate can function in a group setting.

2. The child must have the potential to talk about the molestation in group, and must be able to tolerate hearing about other children's experiences without serious acting out.

3. The child must have sufficient ego strength to be able to wait to speak, to follow group rules, and to attend to the group content.

4. A child with significant cognitive impairment or severe reading deficits may experience difficulty in completing group exercises, which may precipitate disruptiveness, aggressiveness, or withdrawal.

5. Children who manifest psychotic symptoms or are severely depressed or schizoid often do not participate successfully in group treatment.

There are additional factors that therapists should consider, but that do not necessarily preclude group treatment:

1. Children who either deny or greatly minimize their sexual victimization present special problems. These reactions are understandable (and common) in the face of the overwhelming trauma of sexual abuse and the response of significant others. However, the persistence of denial can undermine group cohesiveness and lead to disruptiveness by or scapegoating of the denying child. On the other hand, support from other children with similar experiences can often help to erode denial and to decrease the need for minimization and distortion.

2. Children can be reluctant to participate in group, due to anger at their parents/caretakers for presenting the sexual molestation as the only issue to be addressed in treatment. In these cases, the children feel revictimized, as their sexual abuse is rationalized to be responsible for their families' dysfunction. Where denial and reluctance are strong, individual therapy prior to or concurrent with group therapy is indicated. Denial or refusal to discuss their sexual abuse is especially prevalent among latency-age boys and is addressed in later sections of this manual.

SELECTION OF CARETAKERS FOR GROUP

Caretaker variables must also be considered in the family screening process:

1. Caretakers with severe psychopathology, untreated substance abuse, or a history of severe child neglect are not suitable for inclusion in group. These adults often are either totally unable to listen to and empathize with

others or become debilitated between sessions because they "take on" the problems of others.

2. Caretakers who completely deny that the abuse occurred, in spite of preliminary individual and conjoint treatment, should not enter group. In these cases, group cohesion and goals are inevitably undermined by the formation of cliques, and a sense of despair can develop when other group members attempt unsuccessfully to confront the denial.

3. Caretakers who are highly ambivalent about believing their children, and/or remain actively involved with denying perpetrators, may sabotage the treatment because of ongoing loyalty to the perpetrators.

4. Adults with rigid belief systems that do not allow for exploration of issues of sexuality and anger will impede group process.

5. Caretakers who are too enmeshed with their children will find the children's involvement in a separate group experience intolerable.

6. Caretakers who have tremendous anger about their court-ordered status may not be able to develop a trusting relationship with other group members or the therapists.

7. Severe marital discord between caretakers is likely to detract from the group's agenda. In these cases one caretaker can be selected to join the group.

8. Foster parents with insufficient emotional investment in a child should not be expected to participate in the adult group. Instead, they can be followed in regular collateral visits to keep them informed of the child's experience in group.

It is important to emphasize that, in many cases, the variables listed above may in fact be present in a minimal to moderate amount in functional groups, and may not always rule out group treatment for a particular family. However, in other instances, these difficulties are so pronounced that either the child or the adult is unable to function in a group, and group treatment must be denied to the family.

Furthermore, once the group is in progress, individual and situational factors must be constantly reassessed. In some cases, the therapists may even need to ask a family to leave group therapy. For example, families who are habitually absent or tardy, even after repeated warnings, must be discharged because this behavior undermines group process. When premature termination is deemed appropriate, it should be done quickly to avoid protracted struggles and the further erosion of group cohesiveness. However, therapists must be prepared for a period of regression following unexpected termination of a group member. This may require a temporary suspension of the curriculum in order to address the inevitable reactivation of feelings of loss and betrayal.

In addition to evaluating individual characteristics, therapists must recognize that the vast majority of caretaker situations are not "cut-and-dried." Increasingly, children are in out of home placement, are in adoptive families, or have recently moved in with a relative or parent. At times, a child will return to live with a non-offending parent from whom he/she has been previously separated, raising powerful feelings related to this relationship that overlay abuse-specific reactions. It then becomes necessary to screen the new caretaker for inclusion. When the therapists are informed in advance that a family is being prepared for reunification, it is also appropriate to include the biological parent along with the current caretaker from the beginning of the program. When a natural parent is found to be unsuitable for group treatment (based on the criteria already outlined), the therapist responsible for that family can instead provide family treatment to ease the transition and address the expected adjustment issues.

The continuing dilemma for the therapists is to juggle the myriad of different caretaker arrangements so that child and caretaker groups can be sufficiently well balanced. For instance, it can be problematic to have only one foster child in a group where the other children are all living at home. Grouping foster parents and natural parents together may also impede cohesion unless a foster parent has had a past history of personal molestation that can be shared with other caretakers. Even in a homogeneous group of natural parents, discordant themes such as the nature of their relationships to the perpetrators and the parents' own history of sexual abuse can retard group cohesion. Each group will require the therapists to stress some issues more than others, providing a sense of security and support for adult concerns. Caretakers must feel safe to bring up any family/personal problems that affect the caretakers' ability to support their children's treatment. The therapists must decide whether adjunct individual therapy will be necessary in order for an adult to function well in group.

While the curriculum in this manual is designed to deal with the sequelae of sexual abuse for both children and caretakers, families usually present with a multitude of problems that cannot be addressed by group therapy alone. At times, families are preoccupied with postdisclosure adjustments that include unresolved legal disputes. In other instances, children present serious symptomatology, such as encopresis, suicidal thoughts, separation anxiety, or oppositional behavior. Caretakers may suffer from grief, depression, major life changes, and financial strain. The group treatment program is not designed to focus on all of the individual problems that families experience. Although staff shortages may interfere, the authors strongly recommend providing individual and family treatment for all group participants. This allows children and caretakers to concentrate more readily on the group curriculum, since they are assured that therapists will also be addressing personal concerns in supplemental sessions.

When adjunct treatment cannot be provided by the group therapists, families can be referred to other treatment facilities in the community. In these cases, regular contact between group and outside individual therapists is essential to share information, to coordinate treatment, to prevent splitting, and to facilitate the attainment of treatment goals.

PREPARATION OF CHILDREN FOR GROUP

Upon completion of the initial screening, an additional two to three individual sessions are necessary to prepare a child for group. The child's anxiety level should be addressed during the preparation phase. While moderate anxiety prior to beginning group is anticipated, severely anxious behavior can impede the child's ability to contribute to and benefit from the group experience. In order to alleviate the child's apprehension, the therapist should explain that all the children in group have similar experiences and feelings. A description of the format and structure of group will further reduce anxiety and give the child a greater sense of mastery prior to entering group. The therapist should present the group rules concerning confidentiality, fighting, scapegoating, and ridicule about having been sexually abused. The child must be reassured that the therapist will be present and will be supportive and protective.

In addition, children should be informed that they will eventually be asked to talk about the sexual abuse experience in group. This may increase anxiety for children who have already had to repeat their story several times and may feel embarrassed to tell it again in front of peers. Children often express the fear that they will be belittled or disliked by other group members for "allowing it to happen," especially when there has been more than one perpetrator or when the abuse was chronic and severe. This discomfort about disclosure can be reduced if a child is allowed to practice disclosing in the individual sessions and is reassured that the uncomfortable feelings evoked by this discussion are normal. Of course, children can also be reassured that they are not expected to share their experiences until they develop trust and feel comfortable with the other group members.

Along with those areas of preparation already discussed, male victims of sexual abuse challenge the therapist with an additional set of concerns. Sexually abused boys frequently have a history of poor peer relationships due to hyperaggressive behavior, and enter group with a high level of anxiety about whether they will be liked by the other group members. Those boys who have assumed a more passive stance may fear revictimization. A description of the group to prospective members must stress the importance of being with other boys and learning how to make friends, thus appealing to their need for involvement with male figures.

For boys, the most common issue during the preparatory period is the reluctance to discuss the sexual abuse in front of peers. Boys are encouraged to enter into a "contract" with the therapist, agreeing to full disclosure once they become comfortable in group. The contract actually makes group disclosure easier for boys; they feel empowered after they promise to take this active part in their own recovery. The therapist may decide to allow a boy into group who is unable to make this contract if it is anticipated that the atmosphere of the group will promote comfort with disclosure by reducing his sense of isolation and stigmatization.

PREPARATION OF CARETAKERS FOR GROUP

It is equally important that there be a preparatory period for the caretakers. During these sessions, more detailed descriptive and historical information regarding child and family difficulties is reviewed. The therapist should attempt to clarify the preabuse functioning of a child and family, and to assess the impact of sexual abuse and disclosure on all family members. Caretakers should be helped, as part of this process, to specify some concrete goals for themselves as well as for their children. This is also the time to evaluate the emotional adjustment and functioning of siblings, including their knowledge about and response to the victim. If possible, individual or group intervention should be offered to these children as well.

In preparing caretakers for their own and their children's group experience, it is also important to explore their concerns about confidentiality. In addition, it is critical that caretakers understand the therapist's expectations regarding the nature and consistency of their participation. The primary vehicle for accomplishing this task is the written agreement (see end of chapter for a sample contract). This should include clear statements regarding the need for consistent attendance, criteria for premature termination, an explanation of the limits of confidentiality with regard to the courts and protective services, and a general description of the content and structure of both child and caretaker groups.

Caretakers experience a number of common anxieties before group entry. Natural parents often anticipate being blamed by other group members and/or the therapists for the sexual abuse. This fear, born of their own sense of guilt, is often well hidden, manifested through the use of hostility and cynicism.

Many caretakers are concerned that the experience of group will be too upsetting for the children and worry that their children will be revictimized by having to talk about the sexual abuse in group. "Putting the experience behind them" is often perceived as the best course of action. With these families, the therapist should stress the importance of exploring feelings related to the abuse in a group setting while empathizing with caretaker concerns. Caretakers can be told that "forgetting" without exploring and integrating the experience may lead to future problems, such as sexualized behaviors and depression. Families do suffer a great deal by the disclosure of sexual abuse, and this should not be minimized.

The most commonly expressed concern of caretakers is that their children will hear about more devastating abuse experiences which will adversely affect the children, increasing trauma and preoccupation with the abuse, and influencing future attitudes toward sex. Caretakers fear that sustained attention paid to their children's sexual experiences will make these experiences "too important." Frequently this fear is an indication of the caretakers' discomfort with sexuality and anxiety about their own strong and perhaps overwhelming feelings of rage, guilt, and fear. This is especially salient for those caretakers who have themselves been sexually victimized. Caretakers also express concern that a child's anger or sexually provocative behavior will be stimulated as a result of group treatment. With all of these concerns, the therapist should attempt to convey confidence and assurance that limits and containment are essential parts of the group and that the therapist's role is to make exploration of the abuse therapeutic, not traumatic. However, caretakers must also be prepared for the inevitable manifestations of distress that most children experience as they begin to acknowledge and address interpersonal conflict. It is important to provide reassurance that this discomfort is an expected precursor of a child's growth.

In addition to concerns about the effects of group on their children, caretakers are often quite anxious about their own participation. It is common for caretakers to be isolated, with little or no consistent support system. They may fear rejection by other group members. For others, there is a great sense of relief at finally being able to obtain some support. The therapist should reinforce the caretakers for willingness to take a risk in spite of misgivings about joining the group.

There are also a number of caretakers who see no reason for a parallel adult group and are angry over being made to participate as a condition of their children's treatment. They believe that the therapist is being unreasonable by requiring that they attend group also. While these parents are often overextended (and usually single parents), the therapist must keep in mind that such resistance can be defensive in nature.

Group participation is just as anxiety provoking for adults as for children. During this preparatory period, the therapist should lend support and understanding of the underlying concerns frequently experienced by caretakers. However, resistance to group is often reduced only after caretakers start the group and begin to experience some value in it. Caretakers who continue to be largely "inconvenienced" by the demands of group participation will usually isolate themselves and can undermine group process by continued expressions of anger about the evils of "the system," forcing them to attend group therapy and monitoring their progress in treatment. While there is a place for discussion of such real feelings, the therapists should not allow it to dominate the tone of the group. This issue is discussed more fully in the treatment curriculum; however, therapists should be aware of the possible repercussions of such resistance during the preparatory period.

SUMMARY

Although it is impossible to screen out all potential "treatment failures" before they actually begin group, it is important to pay attention to certain adult and child variables that may preclude successful participation or completion of the goals in the group treatment program. Careful preparation of children and adults prior to group entry can enhance their adjustment and experience in the group process.

However, therapists can anticipate an inevitable phenomenon that occurs in all caretakers' groups, despite careful preparation. At some point, many of the adults will begin to express much anger toward the therapists and to question the value of treatment. It is as though the caretakers perceive themselves and their children as victims. Although this defensive behavior can emerge at various times throughout the group, it is most likely to occur when formal discussion about the molestation begins. Exploration of the conditions under which the abuse occurred often results in a strong reaction in both parents and guardians as they begin to assess ways in which they could be more protective in the future. This attempt to empower the adults can produce resistance and anger, with enormous regression in the face of this unwanted responsibility. The therapists' efforts are experienced as direct criticism, and the caretakers must then protect themselves from the overwhelming sense of guilt by either attacking the therapists directly or insisting that too much is being asked of their children. It is important for therapists to understand the power of the transference even in a structured, directive program, and not to view their efforts as a failure. Fortunately, much of the hostility does eventually diminish with continual validation of the caretakers' difficulty in moving beyond the victim role.

Finally, therapists should never underestimate the profound impact of any change of group leaders, which sometimes occurs in an agency setting. For many of these families, the leaving of a therapist recreates past experiences of betrayal and abandonment, and the inequality in the therapeutic relationship becomes more pronounced. When planning for groups, it is advisable to consider student schedules in order to minimize group disruption.

CARETAKER CONTRACT FOR GROUP TREATMENT

_____ (Name of child)

I, _____(parent/guardian), agree to the conditions for participation in the Children's Sexual Abuse Group Treatment Program as listed below:

1. I understand that it takes 8–10 months to complete the Sexual Abuse Group Treatment curriculum. I agree to participate with my child for at least a 4-month period to determine if group therapy will be helpful to us. During this time, the therapists will evaluate our participation and assess the benefit of group for our family.

2. The groups will meet weekly from _____A.M./P.M. to _____A.M./P.M. on _____(day of week), and my child and I will make every effort to attend all group sessions and to be on time.

3. While an occasional absence due to illness or a planned vacation may occur, I understand that frequent cancellations (more than _____ out of _____ sessions) will result in discharge from the program. I also understand that the attendance rules apply to the caretakers' group as well as the children's group. If it does become necessary to cancel or to be late to a session, I will notify the therapists before the session.

4. I understand that the information shared in the children's group is confidential. However, I will have the opportunity to meet with the therapists of my child's group at least once every 4–8 weeks for feedback about my child's participation and progress in the group. In addition, the therapists in the caretakers' group will provide information about the issues that will be addressed in the child's group to prepare me for possible reactions of my child following a group session.

5. While the therapists encourage my child and me to communicate more openly with each other, I realize that my child may not want to tell me about what happens in group. I will respect my child's need for privacy. I will also protect the confidentiality of other group members by sharing my own experience in the group and not relating what other specific group members have said.

6. I understand that if my child's symptoms worsen or new problems arise, efforts will be made to provide additional individual or family sessions as a supplement for group.

7. I understand that the therapists in the children's and caretakers' groups communicate with each other on a regular basis and that information about what happens in the group sessions is exchanged.

8. I understand and accept that the main purpose of the caretakers' group is to further my understanding about what has happened to my child and its effect on the development and functioning of my child. New knowledge and the opportunity to explore my feelings will increase my ability to support and help my child.

9. I understand that some of the topics discussed in the caretakers' group may elicit painful personal feelings. While the group is an appropriate place to discuss these feelings, it is not uncommon for group members to desire individual therapy. The group therapists can provide referrals for personal psychotherapy and at times may recommend these services.

10. Finally, I acknowledge that all the therapists are required by law to report any new incidents of suspected child abuse as disclosed by either children or their caretakers. In addition, if I am court-ordered for treatment, the therapists will be requested to provide information to the Department of Children's Services or the court about attendance, participation and progress in treatment, and I will be informed about these reports.

Date

Date

Parent/Guardian

Parent/Guardian

Witness

CHAPTER TWO | General Guidelines for Structure and Format of the Groups

A structured group treatment program for sexually abused children and their caretakers provides predictability and establishes boundaries, creating an atmosphere of safety and trust. The curriculum has been designed to address salient issues in sexual abuse that require therapeutic intervention. While it is recommended that all of the modules be completed to achieve the treatment objectives, it is essential to continually assess the needs of group members and their capacity to be receptive and benefit from any particular module. The modules have been arranged in an order that has proven effective but can be modified. In many cases, the themes presented will overlap from session to session, and the therapists can use these opportunities to make connections and reinforce important concepts.

The activities in this manual have been created to facilitate recognition and expression of individual feelings in both children and adults. However, at times the children or adults may respond to an exercise with increased anxiety and resistance. When this occurs, it is best to explore the source of discomfort before proceeding. When the anxiety escalates in the children's group it is usually manifested in disruptive behavior, making it impossible to continue the group discussion. In this case, it is helpful to stop the activity, and allow the children to have some time for free play, or an organized group game. Once the children's reactions have been acknowledged and they are ready to proceed, the therapists may choose to reintroduce or delay the activity or module. In some cases, therapists may acknowledge to the children that they made a mistake by introducing material before the children were ready.

In the caretakers' groups, there will be times when the adults will prefer to present their own concerns/problems and will be resistant to participating in the scheduled agenda. In all cases, therapists must be flexible, attend to the special needs of the children and their families, and be prepared to reorganize and reprioritize the curriculum. However, in order to maximize the efficacy of the treatment, there are definite guidelines that should be followed in both children's and caretakers' groups, to promote consistency and offer a sense of direction for the therapists and the participants.

THE CHILDREN'S GROUPS

The following are important considerations when planning and conducting the latency-age children's group:

1. Same-sex groups are best suited for group intervention with latency-age children, because such groups result in less overstimulation and distraction, and they promote the development of intimacy with same-sex friends. For boys who are dealing with fears and confusion about sexual identity, a boys' group also helps to solidify their sense of maleness, which is often perceived as damaged due to their sexual abuse.

2. Group participation is usually best facilitated with a maximum of eight children per group. This number protects the group against unexpected attrition but is manageable enough for productive interaction.

3. It is advisable to have two therapists in each group. This allows for shared responsibility for the families, the simultaneous use of both psychodynamic interpretation and behavioral interventions (e.g., time out), the opportunity to model cooperative interaction, and, most important, collegial support and feedback. This arrangement also increases the likelihood that group sessions will not have to be canceled in the event that one of the therapists is absent. It is also advantageous to combine an experienced group therapist with a student, in order to maximize staff time and provide training.

4. In recognition of the importance of gender identification for latency-age children, and in consideration of the sensitive nature of the material, it seems best, whenever possible, to use female therapists in the girls' groups and male therapists with the boys. While the addition of a female adult in the boys' group may lead to more cooperative behavior, it may also detract from the camaraderie that occurs with just "the guys." The inclusion of a male adult in the girls' group can be more disruptive when concerns about safety and security result in extreme guardedness or heightened activity to mask anxiety. On the other hand, the gender of therapists in the caretakers' groups has not been a critical factor in treatment success.

5. The curriculum has been planned and organized for a closed group and completion of the program takes approximately ten months. The actual number of sessions and amount of material covered will depend upon the interest and cohesion of the children's and the caretakers' groups. The ending of group should also coincide, if possible, with the schedule of trainees so that the group program will not be disrupted by the inevitable departure of some therapists. The opportunity for the children to experience the group intact from beginning to end is most desirable as it allows for maximum group cohesiveness and promotes a sense of mutual commitment as well as individual accomplishment.

6. The group meets every week for 90 minutes and it is essential that sessions begin and end *on time*, regardless of tardiness or absenteeism. This reinforces the concept of structure and limits and places an important expectation on the caretakers to assume responsibility for their children's treatment.

7. Attendance is acknowledged by recording it each week on a chart where children select and place colorful stickers next to their names.

8. Group rules are developed early, with input from the children. The rules always contain confidentiality and safety requirements but may include a variety of guidelines about cooperation, mutual respect, and expected social norms. While this exercise does establish appropriate boundaries and a sense of empowerment, the children often tend to be overly strict and unrealistic in their expectations. The therapists must help moderate these proscriptions and bring the rules into the realm of realistic compliance.

9. Children are expected to dress age-appropriately for group. This is often an issue for girls, who may come to sessions in provocative attire. It is not unusual to observe a girl strutting in very tight shorts and halter crop top or wearing a blouse so large that it keeps slipping off the shoulder, requiring the child to adjust it constantly throughout the session. In this population, it is important for therapists to address sexualized cues which are often subtle, nonverbal, and out of the child's awareness.

   At times, other group members will comment on a particular child's clothing (e.g., "I can see right up your skirt"), providing an opportunity for therapists to encourage the children to examine their discomfort. In other cases, it is advisable to meet privately with a child to discuss how clothing is selected. It is also important to include the caretaker who may unknowingly encourage the child's behavior. The authors do appreciate the importance of fashion and acknowledge that modern clothing styles can be quite revealing. However, the concern is that girls may use the clothing inappropriately to attract attention to their bodies, putting them at risk of promiscuity or revictimization.

10. A brief snack period is incorporated into the group because of the symbolic importance of food to these children who are often deprived of parental nurturance. Refreshments should be served at the beginning of the session to eliminate any concern that food is somehow contingent on participation in group. The children may even choose to take turns providing the snacks for each other, which helps them feel that they are making an important contribution. Snack time gives the children the opportunity to reconnect and can be used for general discussion about past or upcoming events or anything the children wish to share with the group. Sometimes important information is elicited and the therapists may choose to focus on that instead of the scheduled agenda.

11. The final 15–20 minutes of group are reserved for free play. This allows the children to attain some emotional distance from the difficult work of the group and to interact in a more natural way with peers.

12. Termination of group is presented to the children as a success. They have completed the curriculum and are ready to move on, even if additional individual or family treatment is indicated. A party is held on the final day of group as a celebration of their accomplishment. At that time, each child is given his/her folder containing all the activities (worksheets and drawings) and attendance stickers that the child has acquired during the course of group therapy.

THE CARETAKERS' PARALLEL GROUPS

The caretakers' groups are run concurrently with the children's groups and include nonoffending parents and caretakers (relatives, guardians, foster parents). These groups are designed to emphasize and promote current caretaker–child relationships and are not considered to be adult therapy groups. When preparing for these groups, it is important to be aware of the main goals:

1. To emphasize that the caretakers' commitment to and support for their children are essential to the therapeutic success.
2. To decrease the sense of isolation for the caretakers by providing a safe place for them to share problems, ask questions, and receive validation for their feelings.
3. To assist caretakers in working through and integrating the various responses to the sexual trauma and its aftermath, and to help them to separate their own feelings from those of their children.
4. To educate caretakers about the dynamics of child sexual abuse and increase awareness of the underlying motivation of their children's behaviors.
5. To help caretakers to become more empathic, responsive, and nurturing toward their children.
6. To reinforce the parental role and to help caretakers provide adequate protection from the perpetrators.
7. To increase bonding and improve communication between caretaker and child outside of the treatment sessions.

To achieve these objectives, every effort is made to conduct the caretakers' groups in a parallel manner with the children's groups, using the following format:

1. The caretakers' group also meets weekly and runs for 90 minutes at the same time as the children's group.

2. As discussed for the children's group, it is also advisable to have two therapists in the adult group in order to enhance training benefits and maximize therapeutic effectiveness.

3. In order to reinforce the parallel nature of the group experience and present a team effort, it is helpful to have the therapists switch groups during part of one of the beginning sessions. This gives the children an opportunity to meet their caretakers' therapists, and the adults a chance to meet both of the children's therapists and inquire about their children's initial adjustment. The observations made during this exchange can also enrich therapeutic understanding of the caretaker–child relationships.

4. At the beginning of each meeting, the therapists provide feedback about the previous children's group session including the general response to the structured activity. The caretakers are asked to share any noticeable reactions, changes in behavior, or comments made by their children following the last group meeting. These observations are then discussed in the context of the issues/feelings that were presented and expressed in the children's group.

5. The therapists present the main theme that will be introduced in the children's group that day. The caretakers then address that same issue in their own group with a dual focus on the caretakers' own feelings or fears and their anticipation and understanding of their children's responses. When the children are participating in a specific exercise, the caretakers review the materials, gain an understanding of the purpose, and may participate briefly in the same or a comparable activity designed for adults. This often helps to promote group cohesion and increases the caretakers' capacity for empathy. Therapists also encourage the caretakers to consider and prepare for possible reactions by their children, which may extend beyond the treatment session.

6. As the therapists facilitate the caretakers' interaction around the modules and activities of the children's group, information is often elicited which helps direct the focus of the adult session. Whenever possible, the therapists then attempt to connect the various concerns, problems, conflicts, and general questions raised by the caretakers to the original issue that was introduced.

7. Formal feedback about each child's progress in group treatment is provided to the caretakers during scheduled collateral sessions every 4–8 weeks. A therapist from the children's group and a therapist from the caretakers' group meet together with the parents/guardians of each child to review the parallel treatment and explore concerns or problem areas. In addition, a therapist from the children's group should meet alone with each child to examine the child's use of the group and interaction with peers. When the child is already in individual treatment, this feedback can be incorporated into a regularly scheduled session. Otherwise, a separate interview will be necessary. The caretakers are encouraged to contact the therapists between sessions whenever a question or concern arises, and additional collateral sessions are scheduled as needed.

8. Upon completion of the curriculum, the therapists meet with each family once again to evaluate the benefits they have derived from group treatment and to assess the need for further intervention.

PREPARATION FOR GROUP

Therapists must allow sufficient room in their schedules for group planning and feedback. Time should be set aside weekly to:

1. Decide on which activity to introduce.
2. Inform the caretakers' therapists about the intended agenda so they can consider their strategies.
3. Review the previous session and exchange information about members' participation and various issues arising in each group. This allows the therapists to begin to consider the parallel process between caretakers and their children, which influences the group treatment experience. This interchange also increases therapeutic understanding of family dynamics.

It is also advisable for therapists to save some time immediately following the group session to meet with individual group members when emergencies arise or to pursue sensitive issues which have not been adequately addressed during the group time. Cotherapists may also wish to meet together following a session to consider their own reactions to the group process and examine their interventions.

It is most important to appreciate that a comprehensive group treatment program requires careful preparation and evaluation, and the commitment of considerable time, effort, and emotional investment.

CHAPTER THREE | The Curriculum

The remainder of this manual describes the ten treatment modules which serve to guide the therapists through the parallel group process for child victims and their caretakers. The arrangement of the modules can be best understood when divided into three general phases.

Phase I (Module 1, "Welcome to Your Group"; Module 2, "Making Friends"; and Module 3, "Feelings Are OK") focuses primarily on the initial adjustment to the group experience and prepares the group members by creating a context in which to uncover and resolve many painful feelings and conflicts associated with sexual abuse.

Phase II (Module 4, "Telling Each Other What Happened"; Module 5, "Telling the Secret"; and Module 6, "My Family") concentrates directly on the trauma and disclosure of the molestation and its aftermath, exploring the common themes of betrayal, shame, guilt, responsibility, secrecy, protectiveness, and helplessness as they affect the victims, the caretakers, and the family unit.

Phase III (Module 7, "Taking Care of Myself"; Module 8, "Growing Up for Girls"; Module 9, "Growing Up for Boys"; and Module 10, "Saying Good-Bye") moves beyond the experience of victimization toward recovery and addresses self-esteem, self-protectiveness, preparation for puberty, and finally the completion of the group treatment program.

Each module is separated into five (sometimes six) subsections beginning with the "Purpose," which explains the intent of the module, outlines and connects the major issues for both children and their caretakers, and provides the rationale for inclusion and sequential placement of the module. It is important to note that theoretical issues and dynamics are summarized under the assumption that professionals who use this curriculum will already possess sufficient knowledge or will have access to appropriate information about the familiar themes of child sexual abuse and its sequelae. The authors strongly urge therapists who are inexperienced in the treatment of sexual abuse victims to prepare themselves by attending appropriate clinical seminars and reading from the increasingly abundant literature now available.

The "Objectives" section presents the main goals for both children and adults, and although these are separated into specific modules, they are viewed as the general objectives for the entire treatment program. It is expected that some goals may not be reached within the framework of any given module. While the achievement of some objectives may be crucial to the advancement of the group, other objectives may not be accomplished until much later on.

Like the "Objectives," the "Therapeutic Considerations" are not confined to the module where they are first listed. The authors have estimated the circumstances in which each therapeutic consideration is likely to occur but recognize that these issues may emerge at any time. The therapeutic considerations are viewed as expected elements in the group process and are not necessarily negative. They are presented in order to increase the therapists' ability to prepare for and proceed with the curriculum.

In the "Activities" section, the authors establish the number of sessions needed to complete the module and describe how to present each exercise to the children along with the parallel issues to be addressed by the adults. The handouts are provided at the end of each module. The activities are arranged in the order most commonly used by the authors but can be reorganized, repeated, or deleted when indicated. In some cases, the group may develop cohesion so rapidly that some preliminary exercises in the first modules can be overlooked. In other cases, difficulty in trusting, increased scapegoating, or projection may require additional group building, and the therapists may choose to use all the activities in the beginning modules. At times, when there are a significant number of absences, it may be advisable to refrain from introducing a new activity, and therapists can substitute a therapeutic game or engage the members in discussion. At other times, major changes within the group, such as the premature termination of a group member or therapist, may require that therapists repeat earlier activities in order to rebuild group confidence.

An "Additional Resources" section has been included in modules where the use of outside videos, games, or written materials will enhance the curriculum.

In the final section, the authors delineate "Treatment Challenges," which occur frequently and seriously jeopardize the progress of the group treatment, and offer interventions.

The authors believe that this parallel treatment program is extremely useful in assisting child victims of sexual molestation and their caretakers to recover from such a traumatic experience. However, it is important to emphasize that rigid adherence to the curriculum does not guarantee therapeutic success. Healing results from the shared experiences of group members and the quality of relationships that develop over time in group.

Furthermore, a process takes shape in every group that defies structure. Therapists must be prepared for the normal and expected changes in the mood of any group, which alternate between productive interaction and resistance. In addition, particular issues or feelings may emerge at any time, and therapists will need to be creative enough to integrate these issues into the current module.

Finally, progress in group will strongly depend on a variety of external factors, such as premorbid personality structure of the children, degree of family dysfunction, and openness to change. The therapeutic tasks described in the curriculum will be most effective when group interventions are reinforced in the children's homes and are not contradicted or distorted.

MODULE 1 Welcome to Your Group

PURPOSE

The initial sessions of group treatment must focus on the establishment of group norms that facilitate the achievement of the therapeutic objectives. The therapists are responsible for involving the new members in the formation of the group, and for creating an atmosphere conducive to increased mutual understanding, acceptance, and approval. It is important to promote a positive attachment to the group as a unit as well as to the individual members. Successful group treatment requires the development of group cohesion and a safe setting where children and caretakers can begin to communicate their experiences with the therapists and each other. This module also provides the first opportunity to examine group composition and to identify and assess individual social skills. These assessments can be used in conjunction with the structured program to help guide the therapists' interventions.

OBJECTIVES

1. Define acceptable behavior of group members and introduce a respect for boundaries.
2. Promote group interaction and reinforce cooperative efforts.
3. Introduce and encourage the discussion of common experiences to reinforce a feeling of togetherness and promote group cohesion for both children and caretakers.
4. Improve self-esteem through validation of individual feelings and ideas, acknowledging each member's importance in contributing to the group experience.
5. Help group members to understand the purpose of the group.
6. Enhance caretakers' capacity to begin to view their children with increased sensitivity, understanding, and empathy.

THERAPEUTIC CONSIDERATIONS

The therapists can anticipate the emergence of a variety of clinical issues that will greatly influence the success of the group experience. Although many of these issues surface early in the treatment, it is expected that they will continue to exist in various forms throughout the life of the groups. It is important for group leaders to be aware of potential discordant variables which can markedly impact on the direction of the group process. In the initial phase of treatment, the therapists should:

1. Clarify the group purpose in order to address the group members' concerns about direction, limits, protection, and trust.
2. Allow the group to evolve its own identity within the framework of a preimposed structure.
3. Recognize the role of the therapists as social reinforcers through the modeling of cooperative interaction.
4. Establish the guidelines for providing feedback to group members about effective interaction while preparing to transfer this task to the group.
5. Engage the group members in active participation while respecting their need to be cautious, even distrustful, in light of their experience of betrayal.
6. Find a balance between reinforcing commonalities and respecting differences.
7. Anticipate confusion about the relevance of the structured group activities.
8. Reinforce self-protectiveness by encouraging a delay in full disclosure while being sensitive to group members' need to "tell what happened."
9. Understand the complexities of introducing educational material within a psychodynamic framework.
10. Recognize that the members are entering the group experience at different stages following disclosure, which may influence their capacity to utilize the treatment.
11. Anticipate the testing of the therapists' ability to limit aggressive impulses and provide a sense of protection in the children's group.
12. Expect that it will be difficult to shift the focus in the caretakers' groups between child-centered and adult-centered issues.

ACTIVITIES FOR MODULE #1 (3–4 sessions)

1. Introductions

At the beginning of the first session, the therapists make a general statement about the purpose of the group, such as: "This is a place where children who have been molested can come together, and have a chance to talk about what happened to them and find ways to feel better." It is important to state this explicitly, because the beginning exercises do not deal directly with the abuse and, despite careful preparation, children may become confused about the reason for their participation. The therapists can also add that group is a place to learn ways to protect themselves and to make new friends. Therapists should also review the general structure of the sessions.

The children are then asked to introduced themselves to each other, stating their name, age, school, and perhaps some favorite activities. They can also offer their ideas about what they hope to gain from the group experience. Finally, in order to reinforce the intent of the group, the children are also asked to tell who molested them. This request may appear to be inconsistent with the curriculum's intent to allow children to develop trust and comfort before they are asked to reveal such personal information. However, this early disclosure actually diminishes anxiety and promotes the beginning of group cohesion, as it provides concrete confirmation that each group member does share a similar experience. The authors have never observed any resistance to this exercise. In only one case, a girl requested that the therapist tell the group the identity of the perpetrator. This technique can also be helpful in all phases of the curriculum, as some children feel more comfortable when therapists or other group members initially present the information for them.

In the caretakers' group:

> **a.** The therapists review the caretakers' contract and the general format for the group, emphasizing the parallel nature of the treatment program.
>
> **b.** The adults are asked to introduce themselves and discuss what they hope to gain for themselves and their children.

2. Group Rules

This exercise was described briefly in Chapter 2 as part of the general format for groups. In the children's group, the members develop their own rules of behavior and determine consequences. The children take turns listing the rules on a large poster board, which can be brought to each session as a reminder. This process promotes the establishment of boundaries and offers the children a sense of mastery and control. In many cases, children will suggest rules that they have difficulty following; when determining consequences, the children tend to be overly punitive, and some modifications will be needed. For example, one girl suggested that breaking a rule should result in a 2-week suspension from group, while other children recommended that a snack be withheld.

In the caretakers' group, the adults:

> **a.** Consider what rules/consequences their children will select.
>
> **b.** Describe how explicit and implicit rules of acceptable behavior are established, communicated, and enforced at home.
>
> **c.** Select rules for their own group, reinforcing the importance of structure and limits. The adults often ask for the same rules as the children, such as "Don't be critical."

3. Group Picture

In this cooperative activity, the children are given a large piece of paper and markers and are asked to make a picture together. They must decide on a theme and assign each other roles for completing the picture. This process introduces the children to the idea of negotiation and is an opportunity for the therapists to observe the different strategies each child applies in an attempt to be a part of the decision-making process. The activity also promotes bonding. In one group, the members agreed on a picture about Christmas, which led to all the children sharing their holiday plans and the presents they hoped to receive.

In the caretakers' group, the adults consider:

> **a.** What roles their children will take in the group activity (e.g., leader, follower).
>
> **b.** How roles are assigned and decisions made within each family.
>
> **c.** How the children/adults view themselves in relation to others (e.g., need for approval, indifference).
>
> **d.** How the adults feel about being in a group. One father stated that he was participating in group because he was "afraid not to be here."

4. Being a Member (Handout 1-1)

This is the first exercise that uses a written handout. (At this point the group members are given their personal folders, where they will collect all of the materials used during the course of treatment. The children are given permission to decorate their folders.) This activity helps the children to compare experiences within their own families to their participation in other group situations. The children are asked to list ways they participate as members of their families (e.g., take care of a younger sibling), their classrooms (e.g., listen to the teacher), and the therapy group (e.g., don't make fun of anyone).

In some cases children will demonstrate difficulty reading the written material. When a child asks the therapists about the pronunciation or meaning of a word, it is usually best to determine whether the rest of the group members understand the word. For group members who have reading or comprehension deficits, it will be necessary for one of the therapists or another group member to assist those children in completing the handouts.

The therapists use the written responses to help the children examine their similarities and differences as members of different groups, and to clarify the children's expectations of themselves and others within the group treatment setting. Like group rules, the expectations about group conduct can be referred to throughout the group treatment, whenever the children begin to demonstrate disruptive or alienating behavior.

In the caretakers' group, the adults address:

> **a.** Their expectations of how their children will behave in different group situations.
>
> **b.** What is acceptable and unacceptable group behavior.
>
> **c.** Personal experiences in groups and examination of how the treatment group experience is unique.

5. I'm Like You . . . I'm Different From You (Handout 1-2)

In this activity, each child is asked to select a category (e.g., first names, movie stars, sports, colors). Once a category is chosen, the child writes it on the top of the handout and takes a turn engaging the group members in completing the handout by finding three items in this category that all the children like, three items that some of the children like, and three items that only one of the children likes. For example, if a child chooses the category "sports," he/she then names different sports out loud and the other group members raise their hands if they like that sport. The child must find three sports that every group member likes, three sports that some members like, and three sports that only one member likes. The children take turns until each child has an opportunity to choose a category and complete the activity sheet. This exercise serves to reinforce similarities while respecting uniqueness. It allows the therapists to explore the children's responses to peer pressure, and permits the beginning expressions of feelings/fears of being different. Most children are delighted to learn that other group members like the same movie stars, cars, or rock bands that they do. However, an occasional child will feel the need to maintain distance from the others by opposing every selection; for example, if everyone else likes hamburgers, this child will "hate" hamburgers.

In the caretakers' group, the adults are asked to participate briefly in the same exercise in order to generate discussion of the following issues:

a. How their children will respond to the exercise (e.g., conform or be oppositional).
b. The caretakers' investment in how their children behave in a group (e.g., do they worry if their children will "fit in"?).
c. The adults' awareness/appreciation of peer investment and approval and how these relate to self-esteem.

6. Learning about Each Other (Handout 1-3)

The children interview each other in pairs, using the structured questions included on Handout 1-3. Time is allotted for each participant to act as both interviewer and interviewee. When there is an uneven number of children, the extra group member can be added to one of the pairs. Once the handouts are completed, the children then take turns telling the group what they have learned about their partners. This activity helps to encourage beginning trust in others, serves as a transition to the second module, "Making Friends," and is used again in a different way in that module. In activities in which children are paired, it is advisable for the therapist to assign the pairings, thereby diffusing cliques and integrating withdrawn children.

In the caretakers' group, the adults:

a. Consider what their children's answers will be to the questions on Handout 1-3.
b. Participate in the same interview format, using a more adult-centered set

of "Interview Questions" (Handout 1-4). This exercise for the adults helps to decrease feelings of isolation through the identification of common interests and experiences. It also serves to engage members who aren't certain that they "belong" in the group.

ADDITIONAL RESOURCES

1. The UNGAME (1975). (Available from The Ungame Co., 1440 South State College Blvd., Building 2-D, Anaheim, CA 92806)
2. The Talking, Feeling and Doing Game—A psychotherapeutic game for children (1973). (Available from Creative Therapeutics, 155 Country Road, Cresskill, NJ, 07626)

These games facilitate group interaction and validate children's feelings.

TREATMENT CHALLENGES

In this first module, the therapists may experience the following problems and resistances:

1. The caretakers may be unwilling to participate in the activities, viewing them as irrelevant and demeaning. When this occurs, the therapists should first determine whether the reluctance applies to all or only a few members and encourage a dialogue between the different viewpoints in order to elucidate the objections. If clarification of the resistance does not resolve the conflict, the therapists can then again review the purpose of the caretakers' group and the value of addressing issues in a parallel way to promote closer alliances between adults and children. Finally, the therapists may need to effect a compromise, in which caretakers will participate in selected exercises and only review the remaining ones. Whatever the resolution, it is most crucial that the adults contribute to the decision-making process.

2. Caretakers may express concern that their children are being "forced to participate" in activities and view the therapists as coercive. Therapists should always reinforce caretakers for their capacity to be protective of their children, but reassure them that the children are never forced to participate in any activity. It is also useful to encourage the adults to explore the feelings evoked when their children complain of being coerced.

3. As the groups begin to evolve, therapists may discover that certain children/adults are not appropriate for this treatment modality, and that their continued participation may be destructive to the group experience for the other members. Therapists must then weigh the positive or negative impact of removing them from the group. In some cases, a few individual sessions may be useful to provide feedback to a group member about

therapists' concerns and to explore ways in which the child or adult can more effectively utilize the group. Adults especially may be able to remain in group with concurrent individual psychotherapy. In other cases, it will be therapeutically appropriate to terminate a family from group, stimulating feelings of helplessness and fears of abandonment by remaining group members. The inevitable erosion of group trust is often manifested in extreme regression and hostility which must be addressed directly by the group leaders. Resistance must be actively interpreted within the context of group members' overwhelming vulnerabilities.

4. Despite the therapists' best efforts to delay in-depth discussion about individual sexual abuse experiences, the children and the adults may suffer increased anxiety about how other group members will respond to their disclosures. This discomfort may interfere with some members' ability to benefit from the beginning exercises. In all cases, the therapists should present the rationale for imposed limits, explaining that people usually find it easier and more helpful to share the details of the molestation and other very personal information after they know the other group members better and have developed feelings of trust. When group members reveal information prematurely, therapists should not actively pursue it, but should acknowledge and empathize with its importance and reassure the members that they will have ample opportunity to talk about these issues in future sessions.

5. Some caretakers express the belief that they have nothing in common with other group members because their children have no symptoms. Therapists must remind caretakers that children who have been sexually molested experience common feelings and conflicts, and without intervention they remain at risk for future difficulties.

Name _____

Being a Member

I do some things because I am a member of:

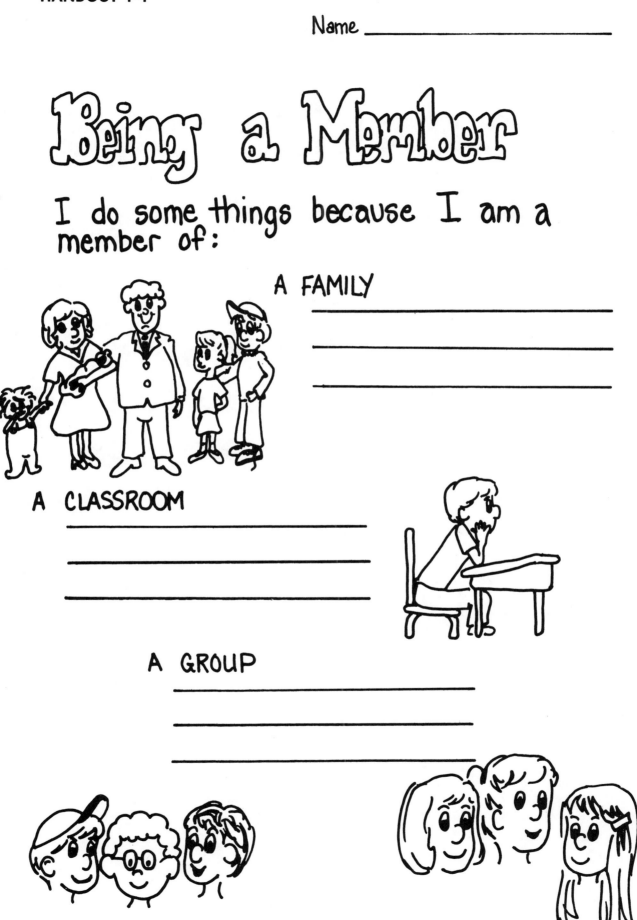

A FAMILY
_____
_____
_____

A CLASSROOM
_____
_____
_____

A GROUP
_____
_____
_____

Name _____

I'm like you ...
I'm different from you

CATEGORY: _____

Everyone in group likes:

_____

_____

_____

Some members in group like:

_____

_____

_____

Only one member in group likes:

_____

_____

_____

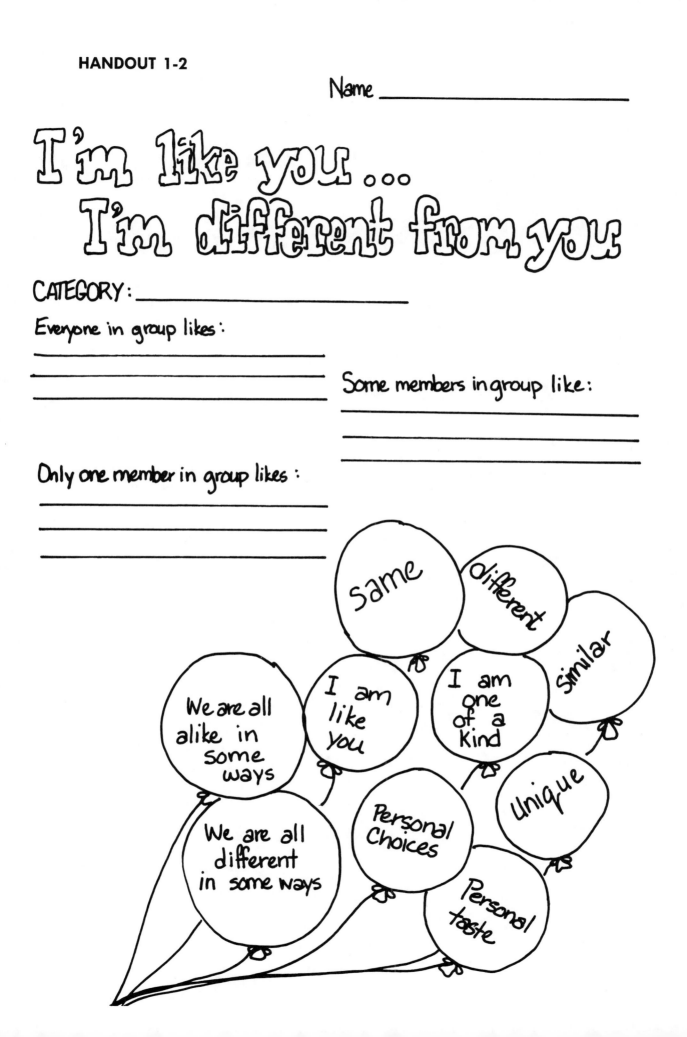

Name _____
Interviewer _____

Learning about each other

1. How old are you? _____

2. Whom do you live with? _____
_____

3. What do you like best about school? _____
_____

4. What are your favorite things to do? _____
_____

5. What kinds of things do you like to do with your family? _____
_____
_____

6. What is your favorite TV show? Why? _____
_____

7. What would you like to be when you grow up? Why? _____
_____

8. If you could have any three wishes, what would they be?
   1. _____
   2. _____
   3. _____

9. What do you like best about yourself? _____
_____

10. What one thing about yourself would you like to change? _____
_____

HANDOUT 1-4: INTERVIEW QUESTIONS

1. Who do you live with? Briefly describe each family member (use 3 words for each).

2. If you could have a day all to yourself, how would you spend it?

3. If you could choose any career, what would it be? Why?

4. What is your best quality?

5. What qualities in your personality do you see in your child?

6. What makes you a good friend?

7. Who is your best friend? Does that person know that your child was molested?

Complete these sentences:

8. I hope this group will help me to better understand
   _____ about my child.

9. I hope this group will help me to better understand
   _____ about myself.

MODULE 2 Making Friends

PURPOSE

This module focuses on the continued development of group cohesion and trust while highlighting the establishment of peer relationships. The most salient feature of latency is the increasing investment in one's own peer group and the acquisition of those social skills necessary to build satisfying friendships. As previously discussed, children who have been sexually abused feel somehow different from their peers. In addition, group members frequently experience difficulty making decisions about whom they should tell about their sexual molestation. Some children are so fearful of being discovered that they avoid peers, while others show very poor judgment by telling many people and inviting ridicule. This module continues to aid in the development of trust, to promote and reinforce mutually supportive peer interactions, to explore feelings of being damaged, and to assert the importance of appropriate boundaries in peer relationships. In addition, the adults are encouraged to gain understanding of their children's anxieties and to evaluate the nature of their children's friendships, which is a prime area of concern for caretakers who have meager support systems and feel embarrassed about their children's sexual abuse.

OBJECTIVES

1. Promote positive peer interactions in the group setting.
2. Strengthen the growing trust among group members.
3. Clarify and allow for the expression of feelings of stigmatization.
4. Reinforce group members' ability to establish criteria for the selection of friends, thereby increasing a sense of personal power and worth.
5. Explore children's and caretakers' anxieties regarding who should be told about the sexual abuse, and evaluate the possible consequences of disclosing or not disclosing to others.

THERAPEUTIC CONSIDERATIONS

To facilitate the goals of this module, group leaders should:
1. Recognize that the activities in this module can result in the formation of cliques in both children's and caretaker's groups.

43

2. Protect those children who remain in the victim role by allowing other group members to take advantage of them.

3. Anticipate that group members will use each other as targets for displacement and projection. For example, a quiet child may be viewed as "bored" or as "not caring" about the group. In other cases, children often displace rage at the perpetrators onto an oppositional child.

4. Accept that children and their caretakers may be angry with each other because of their disclosure of molestation to friends or relatives.
   a. Strike a balance between a child's need to be protected from intrusion and a caretaker's need to obtain outside support.
   b. Predict that some children will attempt to lessen their anxiety by disclosing their abuse experience to many people who are unlikely to be supportive.

5. Anticipate that some caretakers will be wary of their children's friendships, fearing inappropriate sexual play. Other caretakers display insufficient anxiety even when a child behaves in a highly sexualized manner.

6. Recognize that although it is important for these latency-age children to begin to transfer their energy from the family to the peer group, this process may elicit discomfort and overprotectiveness from the caretakers.

ACTIVITIES FOR MODULE #2 (4–6 sessions)

1. Learning about Each Other II (Handout 1-3)

This is a transitional exercise linking the first and second modules. The children are paired and are asked to prepare a brief "commercial" about each other, using the interview sheet that they filled out in Module #1. The therapists will probably need to model an enthusiastic example of how to convince the group that someone would make a good friend. It should be made clear that presentations are to be positive and persuasive. The use of words like "commercial" and "sales pitch" help make this activity more enjoyable. Presentations are made to the whole group with the child being described sitting in the "chair of honor." The children are often surprised and delighted that other group members view them in a special way.

In the caretakers' group, the adults:

   a. Examine their feelings about the importance of peer approval to their children and themselves.
   b. Consider the degree to which the entire family feels isolated. Caretakers often admit that they "can't talk to anyone" about the molestation.
   c. Engage in this same exercise to better understand the impact of positive peer experiences on their children's self-esteem.

2. Choosing Friends (Handout 2-1)

Each child is given a handout with questions about how friends are selected. As in previous activities the therapists can divide the children into pairs to complete the worksheet. Group members then take turns answering the questions, and the therapists aid in the exploration of pertinent issues. In response to the question, "Where do you make friends?", children will sometimes divulge having little or no contact with other children outside of school. Group members often describe avoiding others for fear that their "secret" will be discovered. Feelings of being "damaged" arise in response to the question, "Do you choose friends who are like (or different from) you?" Children's perceptions of caretakers' attitudes toward their friendships are explored as well. It is not uncommon for children to express anger at caretakers for being too restrictive following the molestation.

In the caretakers' group, the adults:

- **a.** Consider ways in which they either support or discourage their children's friendships.
- **b.** Explore common anxieties regarding their children's friendships, focusing on fears of revictimization and sexual acting out. One mother stated that she would only allow her daughter to see friends in their home until she knew her daughter was "OK."

3. Friends (Handout 2-2)

This activity focuses more specifically on those qualities that make good friends. Each child's own ability to be a friend is also explored. Responses to these questions often center around issues of trust and can be explored in the context of the profound betrayals these children have experienced. This exercise often evokes feelings of confusion about caretakers' admonitions regarding "telling friends" about being molested.

In the caretakers' group, the adults:

- **a.** Explore the quality of their own friendships.
- **b.** Focus on how their own sense of isolation affects parenting and feelings toward their children.
- **c.** Consider the number and quality of their children's friendships. Many caretakers report that since the molestation, their children have been "losing" friends.
- **d.** Discuss their concerns and preferences regarding who knows, or should know, about their children's molestation.

4. Group Role Plays (Handouts 2-3, 2-4, 2-5)

These exercises offer an alternative way for the children to examine how they feel in different roles (such as a dominant or shy role) in the context of an organized social activity. They also have the opportunity to try out and experiment with new roles.

Each scenario includes one character who has been molested and feels uncomfortable in his/her peer group, especially when interest in the opposite sex is talked about. The therapists select one of the role-play scenarios and assign each group member a part. The children are then encouraged to describe how their characters will feel and behave. For example, one child in the role play might remain very passive, allowing others to dominate, in spite of feeling uncomfortable.

Once all the parts are discussed, the children act out the role play, which can last for 5–20 minutes, depending on how involved the children become in the story. The therapists can then address how the children felt playing each role, placing special emphasis on the experience of the "molested" child. It should be noted that matching a child with a role unlike his/her own personality style promotes tolerance and empathy, thereby enriching the experience.

In the caretakers' group, the adults consider:

a. Which roles, in the exercise, best describe their children.
b. Which roles best describe their own interactions in a group activity.
c. Concerns about how the molestation may set their children apart from others, and ways to decrease their children's feelings of shame and isolation.

TREATMENT CHALLENGES

1. Some children may feel demoralized and worthless because of lack of friends. This can reinforce low self-esteem and prompt defensive acting out, usually in the form of insulting others or becoming physically aggressive. The therapists must set appropriate limits and interpret this reaction as a demonstration of the difficulty these children have in making friends. In one group, a child refused to participate in the "Choosing Friends" activity, and an exploration of her resistance led to the disclosure that she had no friends and was teased at school.

2. The focus on intimate relationships may incite fears of homosexuality, making this module and the group experience itself difficult for many boys. The therapists should allow boys the opportunity to engage in less threatening, more traditional play (such as organized sports or board games) in addition to these exercises. Whenever possible, the therapists should also differentiate the feelings of closeness the boys are experiencing from sexual attraction.

Although the children may not be prepared for interpretations about their apprehensions at this stage of group development, therapists in boys' groups must recognize that these feelings tend to permeate the group process and have a profound influence on interaction among group members. Therapists must be attentive to this overwhelming fear which will be manifested in a variety of ways during the activities. Group leaders are urged to review Module #9 in order to better prepare themselves for the inevitable onslaught of anxiety and acting out behaviors that occur when boys feel the need to "prove" their maleness to others. For example, a boy may bring a nude picture of a woman to group, secretly showing it to members. Other examples of counterphobic behavior are "farting," locking someone out of the group room, telling dirty jokes, using excessive profanity and name calling, and fighting among group members before and after the group sessions. Although many of these behaviors need to be limited and contained, they should be understood as attempts to master overwhelming feelings of helplessness, weakness, and passivity.

In the initial phase of group treatment, therapists can merely comment on the behavior, making statements such as "You really like telling dirty jokes." As trust develops and relationships build the behaviors can be connected with their underlying dynamics: for example, "I wonder if you think boys will like you better if you tell really dirty jokes." At a later stage in treatment, if it is believed that a particular child and the group can tolerate a more direct interpretation, the therapists can suggest, "I wonder if telling these dirty jokes makes you feel more like a man." This kind of interpretation begins to address the profound need to defend against the fear of being homosexual. However, the authors caution that every situation must be evaluated individually. Interpretations of this sort too early in the group process severely erode trust and interfere with the boys' capacity to participate openly in group.

3. Despite the therapists' best efforts, cliques can lead to scapegoating of other children. Group members will announce that they "hate" another child or group of children. Therapists should stress the importance of the group working together and can use the exercises that require pairs to dilute potentially divisive alliances. In addition, the group should continually be brought together through a recognition of common experiences and feelings.

4. Group members may form sudden and intense relationships with each other outside the group, which may hinder group cohesion. Breaches of confidentiality will inevitably arise in these situations. In both the children's and caretakers' groups, therapists should explain the importance of working on issues within the context of group. Intense and exclusive relationships outside group can prevent the group from addressing conflict between members within the therapeutic arena. Therapists should also caution group members that these friendships can fall apart as quickly as they form, and this can lead to increased discomfort in group. While it is clearly impossible to dictate individual group members' behavior outside of group, the therapists can advocate that any extracurricular activities include everyone (e.g., birthday parties).

5. The focus of this module requires more intimacy and disclosure in the group. It is not uncommon, especially in the caretakers' group, for members to unite in opposition to the therapists' agenda. They may see the therapists as intrusive or critical. It is important that this expression of

feelings be understood as displaced affects more appropriately directed toward the court system, protective service agencies, or perpetrators. Caretakers often feel helpless in relation to these perceived authority figures, and group becomes a safer target. It is also quite likely that the adults' mistrust of the group therapists is a manifestation of their own sense of helplessness in relation to significant others. Once again, it is important to relate these feelings of being coerced with those experienced in their relationships with the perpetrators and in their own families of origin.

Name: _____

Choosing Friends

1. Where are some places you can make friends?
   a. _____
   b. _____

2. How do you choose a person to be your friend?
   _____
   _____

3. Do you choose friends who are like you? _____
   How are they like you? _____
   _____

4. Do you choose friends who are different from you? _____
   How are they different from you? _____
   _____

5. Tell about one of your friends:
   a. What does he/she look like? _____
   b. What do you talk about? _____
   c. What do you do together? _____
   d. Other people would describe your friend as _____
   _____

6. How do you let someone know you want him/her to be your friend?
   _____
   _____
   _____

7. What do your parents say about your friends?
   _____
   _____
   _____

Name _____

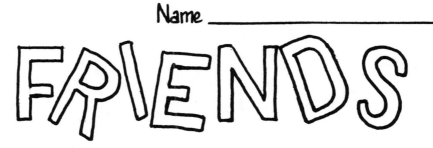

A good friend will:
_____
_____

A good friend never :
_____
_____

I wish my friend would:
_____
_____

I would always tell my friend:
_____
_____

I would never tell my friend:
_____
_____

I am a good friend because:
_____
_____

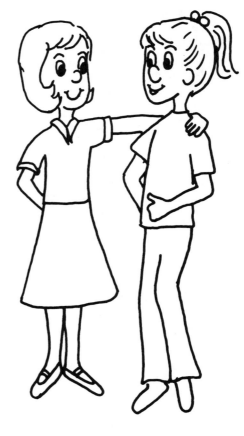

Girls' Summer Camp

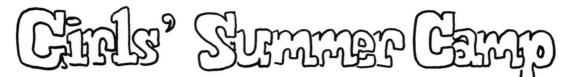

GIRL 1. You act very happy and try to get everybody to get along and have a good time.

GIRL 2. You talk all about your new clothes and can't wait to show off your new swim suit.

GIRL 3. You wish everyone would pay more attention to you, so you interrupt people and try to tell them all the things you are going to do when you leave camp.

GIRL 4. You are kind of bossy and like to tell others what they should be doing. You want everything in the cabin to be neat and clean all the time.

GIRL 5. You don't ever want to change clothes in front of the others, because you feel uncomfortable and worried that someone will be able to tell what happened to you (someone molested you).

GIRL 6. You keep pointing out that there is one girl in the cabin who does not want to change clothes and be like everyone else.

GIRL 7. You ask other girls a lot of personal questions, such as who is in their families and whom they get along with best and where people live.

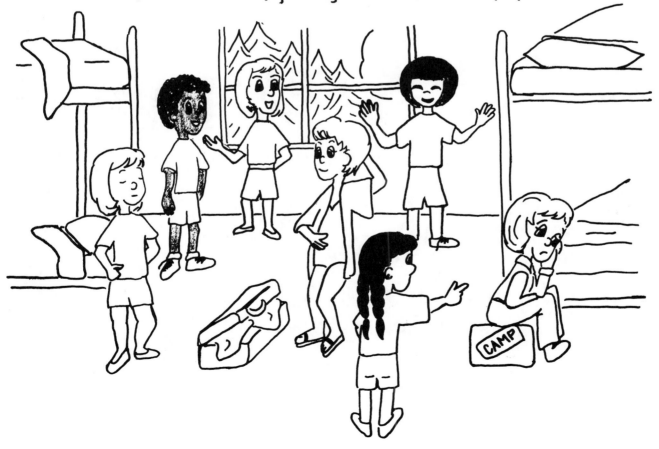

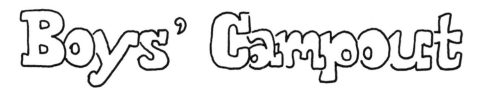

Boys' Campout

BOY 1. You are the boy who wants to know all about the other boys' girlfriends. You ask lots of questions.

BOY 2. You are the boy who has a girlfriend, and you brag to your friends about <u>all</u> the details of what you "do" together.

BOY 3. You are the tough kid who is best at sports and the strongest boy. You think everyone else is a "sissy" and do not believe anything the others say about sex or girls.

BOY 4. You are the kid who does well in school and thinks the other boys are "immature" and stupid for laughing and joking about girls and sex.

BOY 5. You are the boy who really likes camping and would rather tell scary stories by the campfire than talk about girls. You feel that you are too young to have a girlfriend.

BOY 6. You are the boy who has been molested by your uncle. You feel uncomfortable when the boys start talking about girls and sex, so you withdraw.

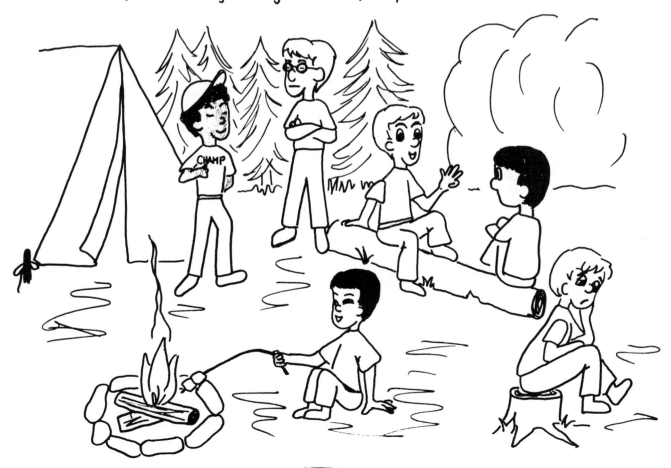

The Slumber Party

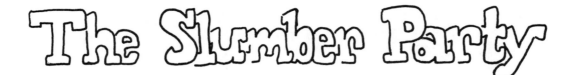

GIRL 1. You are the girl who wants to know all the details about your girlfriends' relationships with boys. Ask lots of questions.

GIRL 2. You are the girl who is having the party. You want all the girls to have a good time.

GIRL 3. You are the girl who has a boyfriend, and you like sharing <u>all</u> the details about what you "do" together.

GIRL 4. You are the girl who thinks that sex is bad and that girls your age are too young to have boyfriends.

GIRL 5. You are the girl who is not impressed with anything anyone says about boys and sex.

GIRL 6. You are the girl who has been molested by your natural father. You feel uncomfortable when the girls start talking about boys and sex.

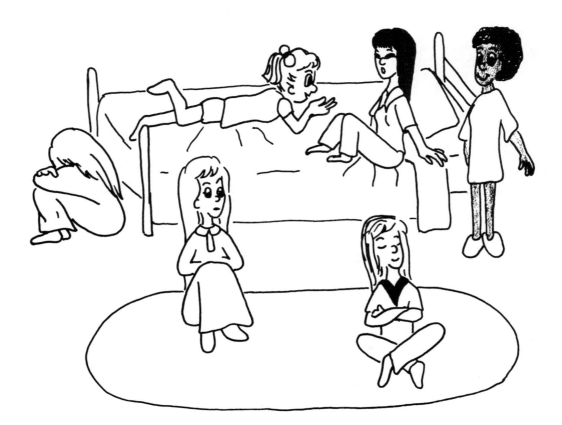

MODULE 3 Feelings Are OK

PURPOSE

This module reinforces the importance of a child's emotional experience and its impact on overall development. Latency-age children often demonstrate a limitation in their capacity to tolerate affect, defending against certain feelings that may be more easily displaced or reflected in overtly manifested behavior. However, acknowledging and expressing feelings is possible for children in this developmental phase. The major therapeutic tasks in this module are to increase the children's awareness of their feelings and assist them to connect various feelings with behavioral expressions. In this way, the acting out of feelings in group will be gradually replaced by verbalization. Caretakers are helped to identify the various feelings that underlie their children's behavior, and empathic responses are encouraged. As the children become more comfortable sharing feelings and concerns, they are ready to move ahead to address the difficult material about the molestation, which will be introduced in the subsequent modules. Finally, this segment attempts to encourage group members to be responsive to the feelings of others.

OBJECTIVES

1. Permit the verbal expression of feelings, thereby decreasing maladaptive behaviors both inside and outside the group.
2. Prepare the children for dealing with a variety of uncomfortable and often conflictual feelings associated with the molestation, such as anger, betrayal, overwhelming fear, sadness, shame, guilt, rejection, and helpnessness.
3. Encourage the development of empathy through the validation of similar feelings among group members, and increase the children's capacity to understand and be supportive of others.
4. Educate caretakers about the impact of emotions on behavior and the ways in which "hidden" feelings can interfere with functioning and adjustment.
5. Increase the caretakers' responsiveness to the behavioral "clues" exhibited by their children, and increase the adults' capacity to tolerate strong affect.

59

THERAPEUTIC CONSIDERATIONS

To promote the acceptance of affective expression in this module, group leaders should:

1. Create a balance between inviting the verbalization of feelings and recognizing the children's need to protect newly established defenses.
2. Anticipate the expected anxiety that can surface when a familiar pattern of mastery is disrupted.
3. Expect the caretakers' discomfort with the children's expression of negative feelings (especially anger), which is often personalized and intensifies their own feelings of guilt. Therapists should predict the adults' reactions and reassure them that verbalization of negative affect is a sign of progress.

ACTIVITIES FOR MODULE #3 (4–6 sessions)

1. What Kinds of Things Make People Feel . . . ? (Handouts 3-1 and 3-2)

The children are asked to describe experiences that evoke feelings such as "sad," "angry," or "happy" (Handout 3-1), or more complex feelings such as "embarrassed," "ashamed," or "jealous" (Handout 3-2). After completing each handout, the children then take turns generating a master list of experiences for each feeling. Although this exercise allows some initial distance from the children's own feelings and encourages beginning empathy, the children will begin to volunteer personal experiences. Children often identify feelings that explain behaviors the therapists have observed. In one case, a child who was extremely quiet in group wrote that talking makes people feel "embarrassed." Another child stated that "some people feel lonely" when they are eating a snack and no one talks to them.

In the caretakers' group, the adults:

a. Explore the kinds of situations their children will associate with the different feelings.
b. Participate briefly in this exercise, examining the feelings that they would attach to various experiences.

2. Feelings Collages

There are a variety of activities in which the children can learn to identify and understand nonverbal representations of feelings. This can be accomplished through one of the activities below in which collages made with magazine pictures are used to depict specific feelings.

a. Each child is assigned a feeling ("sad," "happy," "scared," etc.) and is directed to make a collage using pictures that illustrate this emotion. The other group members then attempt to guess which feeling each collage has portrayed. Once the specific feeling has been revealed, the child then explains his/her collage, describing how each picture represents the feeling. The other group members are encouraged to offer their own descriptions if they recognize different feelings.

b. The therapists list a variety of feeling words on the board. The children are instructed to make individual collages, choosing at least one picture for each feeling listed. Once the collages are completed, the children write down the feeling represented by each picture and present the collage to the group.

c. In a more sophisticated activity, the collage can be used to compare the feelings that group members usually show to others with those feelings they prefer to keep to themselves. Each child draws a large circle on a piece of paper, placing pictures depicting "acceptable" feelings on the outside of the circle and placing pictures depicting "less acceptable" feelings on the inside of the circle. The therapists can use these collages to help the children to explore internal and external pressures to hide certain feelings. One child put a "sad" picture on the inside of the circle, claiming that she would not be accepted by other group members if she expressed sadness.

In the caretakers' group, the adults:

a. Participate in one of the collage activities, exploring their own capacity to recognize feelings on the basis of nonverbal cues.

b. Discuss their own comfort with expressing emotion openly, and consider which feelings are easier to express and which ones they prefer to keep hidden.

c. Learn about ways in which various behaviors in their children may represent unexpressed feelings.

3. "How I Show My Feelings (Handout 3-3)

In this exercise, each child lists on the handout the ways he/she demonstrates feelings nonverbally. The responses are then used as a springboard to increase awareness of the behavioral manifestations of various affects. One child stated, "I brag about things that I can do when I feel stupid"; another child said, "I take extra cookies when I feel lonely."

In the caretakers' group, the adults:

a. Participate in the exercise "Knowing My Child" (Handout 3-4), in which they list and discuss ways in which their children demonstrate a variety of feelings.

b. Consider ways in which the verbalization of feelings is accepted or discouraged in the home (e.g., how often does a caretaker say, "You shouldn't feel that way"?).

c. Examine what they were taught as children about the expression of feelings and what they hope to communicate to their own children. Many caretakers acknowledge that expressing anger was "taboo" when they were children, and that it often resulted in physical punishment.

4. Empathy Role-Play Situations (Handout 3-5)

In this activity, the children are divided into pairs and, in front of the group, enact different preselected role-play scenarios—or, if they prefer, actual personal events that occurred during the week (e.g., a good friend leaves on vacation). One child describes the event, and the other child reacts to it by attempting to guess the feelings and demonstrating understanding and concern. Following the role plays in which children have practiced empathic responses, the group members explore other ways in which they can demonstrate that they understand and care about each other. This exercise offers an opportunity to assess the children's understanding of and capacity for empathy. In one group, the children agreed that the best way to demonstrate interest is to "look at" the person who is talking. In another group, it was decided that "giggling" would not be empathic. The therapists can help the children determine ways to show empathy, which will help them to be supportive in future sessions.

In the caretakers' group, the adults discuss:

a. How they experience concern or indifference by others.
b. How they make themselves available to listen to their children.
c. How they demonstrate empathy to their children. Parents can discuss the ways in which they try to validate their children's verbal or nonverbal expressions of feelings. Some parents will try to deny their children's painful feelings as well as their own.

TREATMENT CHALLENGES

1. Discomfort with the recognition of feelings (such as the identification of anger in oneself or others) may result in withdrawn or oppositional behaviors as coping mechanisms. These may be more pronounced in boys, who dismiss "all this feeling stuff" as unmasculine. In addition to helping the children connect the various behaviors with the feelings they may represent, the therapists must enforce limits. It is essential that despite acting out, children continue to feel safe. As discussed earlier in Chapter 2, it is also important for therapists to acknowledge and respond to the group's distress, allowing the children a brief period of free play or a return to less difficult material until the anxiety diminishes.

2. An escalation or appearance of symptoms outside of group may result in caretakers' complaints and even threats to terminate prematurely. It is important to prepare the adults and help them to anticipate the children's reactions, and reassure them that changes in behavior are an expected outgrowth of the treatment process and are usually time-limited.

3. The children and the adults may demonstrate increased resistance to group treatment as the work becomes more challenging and more time elapses before the actual discussion of the molestation. Therapists should help the group members to understand their resistance and should reinforce what the caretakers have learned so far and the gains their children have made. Therapists can also encourage the participants to discuss their concerns/fears about "what it will be like" to share information about the molestation.

4. The caretakers may feel victimized by their children's expressions of anger ("Why is he angry with me? I wasn't the one who abused him."), and may view the therapists as teaching the children disrespect ("I could never talk to my parents that way!"). Therapists should explore and validate the feelings of hurt, rejection, guilt, and helplessness that are often experienced by caretakers when children express anger toward them. Parents can be helped to figure out acceptable ways in which their children can be angry with them, so that they can then give appropriate guidelines to their children. It is also important to address the possibility that the adults are beginning to view the children's group as a powerful influence, and fear they are losing control over their children.

Name _____

What kinds of things make people feel . . .

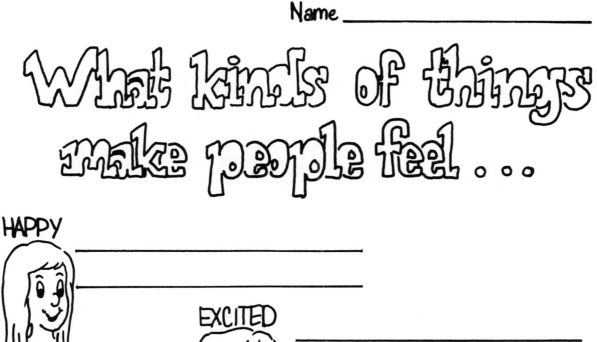

HAPPY _____
_____

EXCITED _____
_____

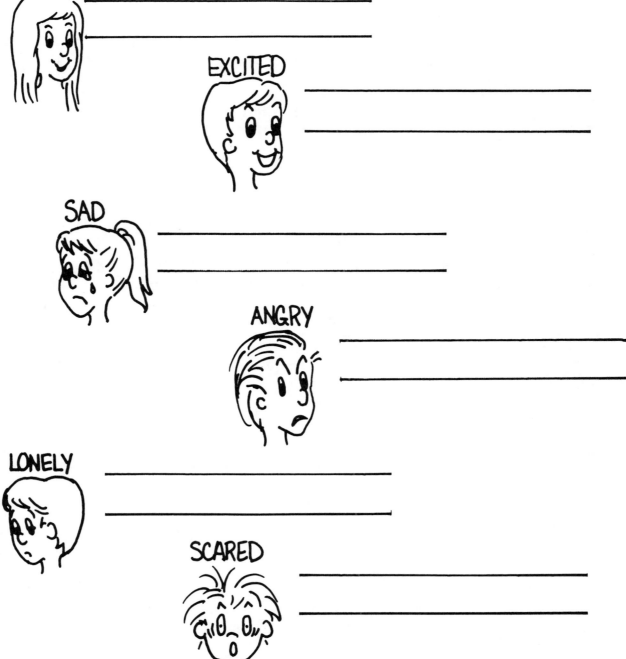

SAD _____
_____

ANGRY _____
_____

LONELY _____
_____

SCARED _____
_____

Name _____

What kinds of things make people feel . . .

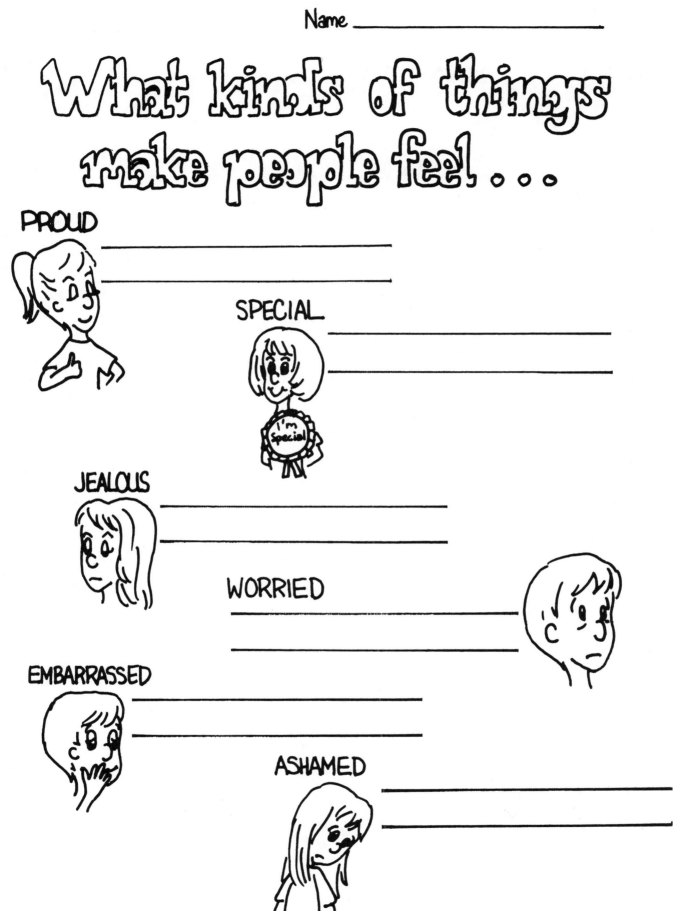

PROUD _____
_____

SPECIAL _____
_____

JEALOUS _____
_____

WORRIED
_____
_____

EMBARRASSED _____
_____

ASHAMED _____
_____

I'm Special

Name_____

How I Show My Feelings

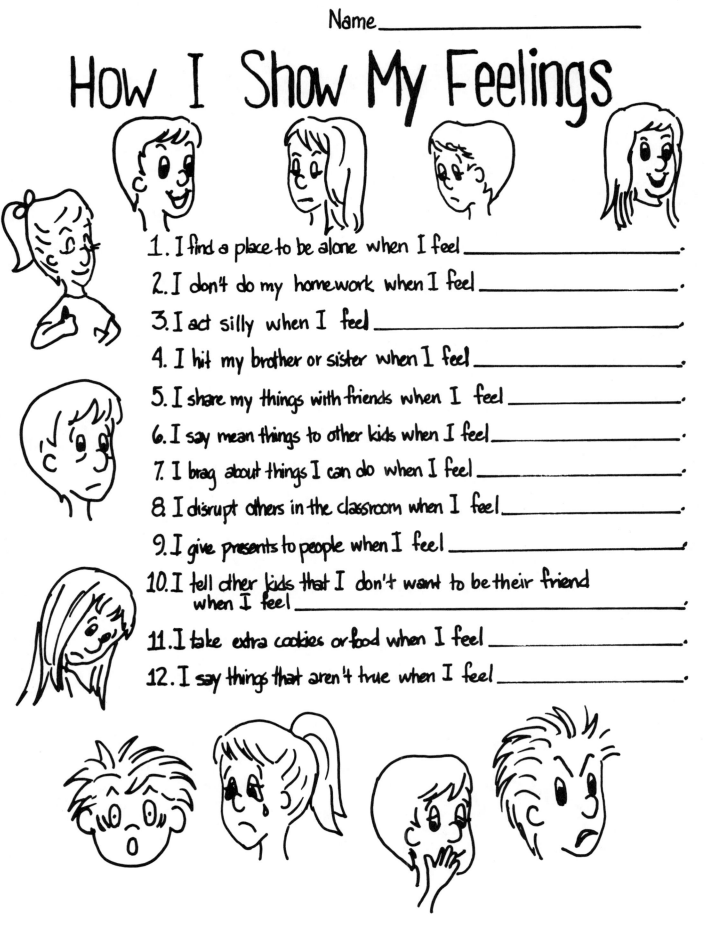

1. I find a place to be alone when I feel _____.

2. I don't do my homework when I feel _____.

3. I act silly when I feel _____.

4. I hit my brother or sister when I feel _____.

5. I share my things with friends when I feel _____.

6. I say mean things to other kids when I feel _____.

7. I brag about things I can do when I feel _____.

8. I disrupt others in the classroom when I feel _____.

9. I give presents to people when I feel _____.

10. I tell other kids that I don't want to be their friend
    when I feel _____.

11. I take extra cookies or food when I feel _____.

12. I say things that aren't true when I feel _____.

HANDOUT 3-4: KNOWING MY CHILD

1. I know my child is worried when _____

   _____

2. I know my child is happy when _____

   _____

3. I know my child is scared when _____

   _____

4. I know my child is angry when _____

   _____

5. I know my child is embarrassed when _____

   _____

6. I know my child is sad when _____

   _____

7. I know my child is jealous when _____

   _____

8. I know my child is nervous when _____

   _____

9. I know my child is lonely when _____

   _____

10. I know my child's feelings are hurt when _____

    _____

Role-Play Situations
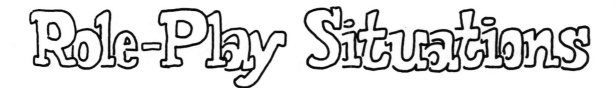

1. My bike got stolen.

2. My mother will not let me go to the movies.

3. I got an "A" on a spelling test that I studied for.

4. I do not know why my brother always picks on me.

5. My parents fight all the time.

6. An older kid made me give him my lunch money.

7. Everybody made fun of me today.

8. I get to go on a trip with my mother.

9. A sixth-grader said he was going to beat me up tomorrow.

10. I have a stomach ache.

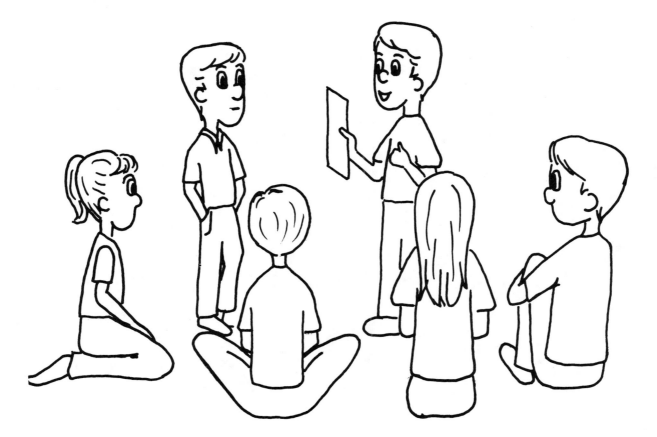

4 Telling Each Other What Happened

PURPOSE

Once the introductory work has prepared the children to identify and express positive and negative feelings, they are ready to focus on their sexual abuse experiences, which will be addressed in a variety of ways for the duration of the group treatment. Until now, the children may have received confusing messages from their caretakers about whether it is acceptable to talk about their molestation. Once the children have disclosed to family members and legal authorities, there is often an external pressure to "put the experience behind them." Some parents do not want to know "all the details," preferring to believe that the molestation was minimal. In other cases, the courts prohibit parents and children from talking about the abuse, and foster parents and guardians often discourage the children from sharing the experiences with them. Therefore, this phase of treatment gives the children permission to tell what happened to them and provides support for feelings that are often hidden. In addition, this module begins to consider the positive and negative features of the relationships between victims and perpetrators. The therapists aim to reinforce the children's ability to talk about the molestation and to be supportive of other group members' disclosures as well.

OBJECTIVES

1. Permit verbal expression and validate feelings about the abuse experience, thereby reducing the risk of uncomfortable feelings being manifested behaviorally.
2. Clarify the confusing feelings about the perpetrators for children and caretakers.
3. Decrease isolation and feelings of stigmatization by encouraging the children to share details of the molestation with others who have had similar experiences.
4. Assist the children and the adults in the identification and understanding of feelings of guilt and responsibility related to victimization.

THERAPEUTIC CONSIDERATIONS

In order to facilitate discussion of the molestation, therapists should:

1. Proceed very carefully with the sharing of very personal, often explicit material, respecting the children's and the adults' need for privacy.

2. Anticipate that disclosure may cause some divisiveness even in a cohesive group, resulting in withdrawal or aggressiveness by children who are certain they will be disliked once their story is told.

3. Help the children to differentiate lack of responsibility from powerlessness. Examining what they can do differently in the future reduces the risk of further victimization.

4. Attend to the details of disclosures, because new and potentially reportable information may be revealed.

5. Realize that the trust and cohesiveness of the caretakers' group will be profoundly affected if a caretaker reveals that he/she is a child molester.

6. Keep in mind that there may be developmental limitations in younger latency-age children that interfere with their understanding of the concept of ambivalence. Some children may have difficulty accepting that it is possible to have both positive and negative feelings toward the same person.

7. Help caretakers who were molested as children to separate their own feelings from those of their children.

8. Anticipate that some children and caretakers will compare their own or their children's molestation to that of others in group; such comparisons may either reinforce minimization or increase shame or stigmatization. They need to be helped to separate their own experiences from those of the other group members.

9. Help caretakers anticipate highly anxious reactions from their children.

10. Assist parents who have had trouble believing their children to reexamine their feelings at this point.

11. Recognize the profound influence of the caretaker's relationship with and attitude toward the perpetrator on the child's freedom to express his/her true feelings about the molestation.

12. Acknowledge the extremely sensitive issues involved in sibling incest, where caretakers may feel an obligation to support and protect the perpetrators.

ACTIVITIES FOR MODULE #4 (6–8 sessions)

1. Feelings about Being Molested (Handout 4-1)

In this exercise, the children begin to consider the feelings associated with the molestation. On the handout, the children rate the intensity of a variety of feeling experiences. (This is the first of several handouts that designates the perpetrator with a blank space, allowing the child either to write in the name of the perpetrator or to use the appropriate pronoun, "he" or "she.") The therapists then help the children to identify and examine the feelings described. For example, responses to the statement "I thought

_____ really did care for me" can lead to a fruitful discussion about ambivalence toward a molester, who is often viewed as the more nurturing caretaker. It is important for therapists to reinforce commonalities but to acknowledge that each child's experience may be different, depending upon external and internal circumstances. It may also be useful to reintroduce this activity at the end of the group experience, in an effort to examine how the children's feelings about being molested may have been affected by the treatment.

In the caretakers' group, the adults:

- **a.** Discuss how they think their children will respond to the activity sheet.
- **b.** Examine their own feelings about the molestation and how these feelings have changed over time.
- **c.** Consider the most painful feelings that their children experience.
- **d.** Describe ways they encourage or discourage their children to express feelings about the molestation.

2. I Think This Happened Because . . . (Handout 4-2)

In this exercise, the children are asked to list reasons why they think they were molested and reasons why they think the perpetrators did it. The answers are used to help the victims relinquish blame and responsibility while attempting to make sense out of their experience, decreasing the overwhelming feelings of helplessness. Children often think that the perpetrators were "sick" or "crazy," or even "victims"; this may result in "feeling bad" for the perpetrators and reduces the children's capacity to assign responsibility. When group members suggest that the molesters may also have been abused as children, it is an excellent opportunity to explore indirectly the possibility that some group members may have already sexually abused others. Children also search for answers to explain their victimization. One girl believed she was molested because she was "quiet and shy" and the perpetrator must have known she would not disclose; another girl thought she was molested because her father "needed an excuse" to leave the family. Boys often reveal fears that they were abused because the perpetrators "knew they were weak."

In the caretakers' group, the adults:

- **a.** Consider how the children view their victimization.
- **b.** Explore their own ideas about why their children were targeted to be molested.
- **c.** Review their own relationships with the perpetrators and identify feelings of responsibility and blame for the molestation.
- **d.** Begin to examine the possible motivations of the perpetrators.
- **e.** Address their fears that their children might be revictimized or become perpetrators.

3. What Will People Think of Me? (Handout 4-3)

In this exercise, the children complete a handout that addresses expectations and fears of rejection or ridicule once the details of the abuse are revealed. One girl admitted that she didn't tell anyone about being molested by her father because others would think she had a "bad mother." One boy feared others would "blame" him and think he was "stupid."

In the caretakers' group, the adults explore:

  a. Their concerns about how others will respond when their children "tell what happened."
  b. Their fantasies about what others think of them as parents of children who were molested.

4. Telling Each Other What Happened (Handouts 4-4 and 4-5)

The children are paired and asked to interview each other using a questionnaire that asks about each child's relationship with the perpetrator and the details of the molestation. The children are instructed to complete the handout as best they can, and if a question is too embarrassing they can say so. The questions are then shared with one child in preparation for disclosing in group. The opportunity to "practice" can help to reduce anxiety and build trust. After completing the interviews, the group reconvenes, and each child takes a turn sharing his/her molestation experience with the group. In one group, as the children took turns telling the age when they were first molested, one girl became extremely embarrassed and refused to speak. She had been 4 years old when the abuse first occurred, and so far the other group members had been "at least" 8. Her partner, who had been molested at age 2, volunteered to share her age first in order to pave the way for the embarrassed girl.

In the caretakers' group, the adults consider:

  a. How the children will respond to the interview questions.
  b. The feelings that might be elicited in their children by the disclosure to the group.
  c. Whether they feel that their children will be open to sharing the details of the molestation with others.
  d. How they feel about their children disclosing in group and learning of other children's experiences, which may be more or less severe.

5. Letter to the Perpetrator (Handout 4-6)

This activity gives the children an opportunity to begin to confront their perpetrators. For some children, it will be a preparation for face-to-face meetings prior to families' reunification; for others, it may be the only way they can "talk" to the perpetrators. Each child is asked to write a letter to the perpetrator, sharing his/her feelings about what happened and feelings about the perpetrator(s). If a child was molested by more than one person, he/she can write a letter to each perpetrator or select only one. The children are permitted to use strong language (e.g., familiar swear words). They are also encouraged to express any good feelings or memories. Many children demonstrate ambivalent feelings by signing a very negative letter with "love." Other children convey only positive feelings, which may leave them vulnerable to ridicule by other group members or lead to antagonistic behavior toward group members who express anger.

After the letters are completed, the children read them aloud; the therapists provide support and validation for their individual efforts, and again reinforce the diversity of feelings that can occur. If the children are reluctant to read their letters in the group, they may share their letters with one other group member first or ask one of the therapists to read it for them. The children may or may not decide to show these letters to parents or caretakers. In some cases, children choose to tear the letters up into small pieces. This gesture is viewed as an attempt to erase the discomfort and guilt that often accompany the expression of angry feelings and should be addressed by the therapists.

In the caretakers' group, the adults:

a. Compare what their children might want to say to the perpetrators with what they will most likely put on paper.
b. Examine their own relationships with the perpetrators and how these affect the feelings they allow their children to express.
c. Write and share letters to the perpetrators, exploring their own ambivalent feelings.

ADDITIONAL RESOURCES

There are many excellent books, videos, and games currently available that can enhance this module. The following are the ones used most frequently by the authors:

1. Harter, S. (1977). A cognitive-developmental approach to children's expression of conflicting feelings and a technique to facilitate such expression in play therapy. *Journal of Consulting and Clinical Psychology,* 45(3), 417–432.
   This article provides an excellent discussion of younger children's emotional and cognitive limitations in regard to the concept of ambivalence, as well as possible interventions.
2. Sweet, P. E. (1981). *Something happened to me.* Racine, WI: Mother Courage Press.
   This book sensitively identifies the feelings commonly experienced by sexually abused children. The group members take turns reading the book and comparing their feelings to those of the different children represented on each page.
3. *Something about Amelia* [Film]. (ABC Television)
   This movie about father–daughter incest validates the many feelings and the isolation experienced by children faced with this difficult problem. It is

an excellent way to introduce this module to both the girls' and the caretakers' groups.

4. *Play it safe with Sasa.* (Available from SASA & Company, 2008 La Brea Terrace, Los Angeles, CA 90046)
   This game deals with many aspects of the abuse experience. The therapists can preselect the cards that ask specific questions regarding children's feelings about being molested, and the children can begin to address their own experience with some initial distance.

5. Groth, A. N. Burgess, A. W., & Birnbaum, H. J. (1978). A study of the child molester: Myths and realities. *Journal of the American Criminal Justice Association, 41*(1), 17–22.

6. Berry, J. (1984). *Alerting kids to the danger of sexual abuse.* Waco, TX: Word.
   This book provides an excellent examination of the ways in which perpetrators trick their potential victims.

TREATMENT CHALLENGES

1. Therapists can anticipate high levels of resistance even from children who had previously been eager to talk about the molestation. The therapists should validate the feelings and encourage open discussion about the anxiety evoked by the disclosure, which could include fear of rejection or loss of friendships. When children are not able to articulate their discomfort, it may be useful to reintroduce some of the initial group building exercises.

2. Some children, because of embarrassment, fear of retaliation, or the wish to protect a perpetrator or nonoffending caretaker, often fail to disclose many of the details of their molestation experience. Therapists are left in the difficult position of knowing the full extent of the molestation and hearing the children's revised versions being presented in group. When this occurs, the children's wishes must be respected. The therapists should acknowledge that some things may be too difficult to share, and leave room for later discussion either in the group or in an individual session.

3. Sometimes one or more children refuse to divulge any information about the molestation, and this refusal is experienced by the rest of the group members as rejection. Therapists should encourage empathy from others and explore ways to make disclosure easier for such a child. For example, another child can be appointed to read the answers, or the child can go last after hearing other disclosures. If a child remains unwilling to participate, the therapists should continue with other group members' disclosures, conveying the expectation that these children can encourage the reluctant child through their "courageous" example.

4. Caretakers often express worry about, and are sometimes in disagreement with, the therapists' wishes for disclosures in the children's group, because

they are afraid that their children will be exposed to and stimulated by explicit language or descriptions of sexual acts that are more severe than what their children have experienced. Therapists should explore how the caretakers believe this will influence their children, and reassure them that the focus is not on the details of the sexual activities but on the feelings about the experience. Therapists should also address the helplessness that caretakers experience when they believe their children are "learning about sex" outside of the family unit.

5. Conflict may occur among the children when group members differ in their attitudes toward the perpetrators. The children who have difficulty integrating their ambivalence, and who thus deny their positive feelings toward the perpetrators, often ridicule and attack those children who continue to express positive feelings. Other children may displace their anger toward the perpetrator onto other group members and be overtly hostile when negative letters are read aloud. It is important for the therapists to permit and acknowledge the conflicting feelings, helping the children to accept the more positive aspects of their relationships with the perpetrators in spite of the intense feelings of betrayal. In addition, some caretakers may be concerned that their children's feelings about the perpetrators will be influenced by peers and the therapists. Therapists must continue to clarify their roles as facilitators, not indoctrinators, and reinforce their respect for individual differences and needs within the group structure.

6. Caretakers may generalize the abuse experience, warning their children that "no one can be trusted" or "men are no good." These proscriptions interfere with the development of positive relationships outside of the family, and may even inhibit the therapeutic alliance. Therapists must be sensitive to the possibility that the caretakers have themselves been sexually exploited as children or as adults, and help the adults to examine how the trauma of the abuse experience has affected their belief systems in an effort to alter cognitive distortions and negative expectations.

Name _____

Feelings About Being Molested

1. I would like to hide from people so I don't have to talk about it.

    never   almost never   sometimes   almost always   always

2. I want to cry.

    never   almost never   sometimes   almost always   always

3. I should have been able to stop it.

    never   almost never   sometimes   almost always   always

4. I thought _____ really did care for me.

    never   almost never   sometimes   almost always   always

5. I feel like a good person.

    never   almost never   sometimes   almost always   always

6. There was something I could do to stop it.

    never   almost never   sometimes   almost always   always

7. I think _____ had a right to touch me.

    never   almost never   sometimes   almost always   always

8. I understand why it happened.

    never   almost never   sometimes   almost always   always

Name _____

I THINK THIS HAPPENED BECAUSE...

I think this happened to me because
_____
_____
_____
_____
_____
_____
_____

I think _____
did it because
_____
_____
_____
_____
_____
_____
_____
_____

HANDOUT 4-3

Name _____

What Will People Think of Me?

1. When others hear what happened to me, they may think that I _____
_____ .

2. I worry that I am the only one who _____
_____ .

3. If I share some of the things I am scared to say, other kids may _____
_____ .

4. People might think I'm weird if I tell them about _____
_____ .

5. The hardest thing for me to tell about is _____
_____ .

6. I was warned that other kids might say _____
_____ .

7. I worry that if I tell everything that happened to me, _____ will get in trouble.

8. I would feel better talking about this if _____
_____ .

What are they going to think...?

What will they think if I tell them everything?

Name: _____

Read these instructions to your partner: You should only tell as much as you feel you can.
When you are too embarrassed, you can say so.

Telling Each Other What Happened

1. How old were you when you were first molested? _____

2. Who molested you? _____

3. What was it like being with _____ before you were molested? _____
_____

4. Did _____ treat you differently after the molestation began? _____

5. Tell about the very first time you were molested. (What did _____ say to you? How did
_____ touch you? Did you touch _____?) _____
_____
_____

6. After the first time, did _____ keep touching you in the same way, or did it change? _____
_____ How did it change? _____
_____

7. Where did it happen? _____

8. When did it happen? (time of day, certain day of the week, etc.) _____
_____

9. How often did _____ molest you? (once...daily...once a month... every week) _____
_____ And for how long? (once... a few months... longer) _____
_____

10. Where was everyone else in the family while you were being molested? _____
_____

11. Did anyone else see you being molested or know about it? _____

12. Did _____ molest anyone else you know? _____

13. If yes, did you see the other person(s) being molested?
_____

14. How did it feel to tell about what happened?
_____
_____
_____
_____

Name: _____

Read these instructions to your partner: You should only tell as much as you feel you can. When you are too embarrassed, you can say so.

Telling Each Other What Happened

1. How old were you when you were first molested? _____

2. Who molested you? _____

3. What was it like being with _____ before you were molested? _____
   _____

4. Did _____ treat you differently after the molestation began? _____
   _____

5. Tell about the very first time you were molested. (What did _____ say to you? How did _____ touch you? Did you touch _____?) _____
   _____
   _____

6. After the first time, did _____ keep touching you in the same way, or did it change? _____ How did it change? _____
   _____

7. Where did it happen? _____

8. When did it happen? (time of day, certain day of the week, etc.) _____
   _____

9. How often did _____ molest you? (once... daily... once a month... every week) _____ And for how long? (once... a few months... longer) _____
   _____

10. Where was everyone else in the family when you were being molested? _____
    _____

11. Did anyone else see you being molested or know about it? _____

12. Did _____ molest anyone else you know? _____

13. If yes, did you see the other person(s) being molested? _____

14. How did it feel to tell about what happened?
    _____
    _____
    _____
    _____

Date: _____

To: _____

    These are some of the things that I have been wanting to say to you.

I used to think _____

and that you _____ .

Then things changed. After you began molesting me I thought that _____

_____

and I wondered if _____ .

When I think of you molesting me I _____

_____ and I feel _____ .

You are _____ and _____ .

Sometimes when I think of you I _____

_____ . I want to tell you that _____

_____ .

If I ever, or when I see you again I will _____

_____ and _____

_____

_____

_____

_____

_____

_____

_____

                                                       _____

                                                       _____

To: _____

P.S. _____

MODULE 5 Telling the Secret

PURPOSE

Once group members have disclosed the details in group and have begun to address their feelings about having been molested, they are ready to more fully explore the conflicting feelings engendered when such a profound secret is kept over time. For all children, the sense of stigmatization, responsibility, and powerlessness appears to be present; however, the varying nature of their abuse experiences and their relationships to both the perpetrators and the nonoffending caretakers powerfully shape the severity and dominance of these feelings. When a child must also consider fears for personal safety and for the safety of others, loss of love and protection, and the breakup of the family, it is no wonder that this secret is often kept for a very long time.

The children's understanding of the reactions of caretakers to disclosure, as well as the subsequent intervention of the child welfare system, is also explored. Following disclosure, a caretaker often experiences strongly competing demands to support the child while maintaining loyalty for the offender, who may be a spouse or lover; in addition, the caretaker may feel unable to confront someone who is perceived as more powerful and dangerous. The legal system often mandates that children be removed from their homes and that they repeat the details of their experience to many different strangers. In many cases, the children and the adults are no more believed, protected, or validated then prior to disclosures. Finally, some children never tell, and it is only through the actions of others that caretakers learn of the molestation. Therefore, the purpose of this module is to help the children to understand and accept the need they had to remain silent, and to reduce feelings of responsibility for the losses and changes experienced by their families following disclosure. Caretakers are aided in the exploration of conflicting feelings of anger about their children's secrecy, loyalty to perpetrators, and guilt over their responses to disclosure and their perceived inability to protect their children. This module also aims to increase the caretakers' understanding and support of the children's feelings regarding secrecy while enhancing both the children's and caretakers' ability to express fears and concerns more directly and with greater confidence.

OBJECTIVE

1. Support and reinforce the children's disclosure in spite of negative reactions by others, thereby reducing the risk of future "family secrets."

95

2. Increase the children's understanding of their need to maintain this secret, addressing feelings of responsibility, blame, and helplessness.
3. Prepare the children for court appearances.
4. Provide understanding of caretakers' ambivalence about disclosure, and about their children's participation in the abuse.
5. Help caretakers to understand their children's inevitable feelings about not being protected, even in situations where the caretakers believed there was little reason to be suspicious.

THERAPEUTIC CONSIDERATIONS

In order to support children and adults in exploring conflicting feelings about disclosure, therapists must:

1. Validate the children's disclosure of sexual abuse even when significant adults continue to deny or minimize it.
2. Recognize that the discussion of keeping the secret and its ultimate disclosure will often revitalize children's anxieties regarding being believed, discovery by others, and retaliation by perpetrators, especially when threats of harm to the children or others were made.
3. Anticipate that the focus on disclosure may lead some caretakers to reveal their own childhood molestation.
4. Understand how the children's need to protect the nonoffending caretakers may interfere with acknowledgment and eventual integration of feelings of anger and hurt.
5. Recognize that this phase of treatment requires increased support among group members to reduce the shame and embarrassment that emerge when secrets are shared.
6. Anticipate that children may begin to manifest overwhelming anger as feelings of helplessness surface.
7. Realize that disclosures by the children threaten a very powerful loss in families where the perpetrator is the primary nurturing figure. Therapists must work to bolster the nonoffending caretakers' capacity to be more emotionally available, which may require additional family sessions or a referral for individual adult psychotherapy.
8. Recognize that caretakers often feel helpless themselves and experience the same betrayal as their children.
9. Appreciate the ongoing conflict for some caretakers, who are struggling to reconcile the intense anger toward their spouses or lovers with the wish for reunification. When sibling incest has occurred, parents often experience the same intense conflict, especially when the perpetrators are children they rely on for some emotional support.
10. Accept that the therapists may often feel torn between their wish to advocate for a family and their need to report any deviations from court orders. In order to maintain a therapeutic alliance with court-ordered

families, it is crucial that all letters to the legal system be reviewed by caretakers prior to submission, to allow for their input.

ACTIVITIES FOR MODULE #5 (5–7 sessions)

1. Keeping the Secret (Handout 5-1)

In this activity, group members role-play situations in which one or both of the characters are struggling with the conflict over whether or not to "keep the secret." The different scenarios serve as vehicles for the uncovering and clarification of the feelings that often help maintain secrecy, and give the children an opportunity to play out and discuss their ambivalence. Following one role play, a boy admitted for the first time that he was reluctant to tell anyone about his molestation by his grandfather, because "my mom had too many problems and was always sad."

The children are paired and given a role play to practice. Each pair reads a scenario to the group, and the therapists help the group members to consider the questions posed for each scenario. The pair then plays out the situation for the group. The sample role plays in the handout represent a variety of common dilemmas. Therapists may want to use this format to develop additional ones that more closely address specific issues for the members of any given group. Therapists should also be prepared that following these role plays, some children may reveal that they have knowledge about current abuse situations of friends.

In the caretakers' group, the adults:

a. Consider the process their children went through in deciding to tell, thus gaining empathy for the children's struggle.
b. Review possible attempts their children may have made to tell them about being abused.
c. Seek to understand how something so traumatic for their children could happen, sometimes in their own homes and without their knowledge.

2. Telling the Secret (Handout 5-2)

In this activity, the children are given a structured set of questions about disclosure. After completing the handout, the children use their answers to discuss their experiences with all of the group members. They often express shame over how long they kept this secret and are surprised at the similar experiences of the others. One boy sat quietly with his head down and refused to reveal in group how long he had kept his secret. As soon as another group member admitted keeping the secret for 2 years, he volunteered how ashamed he was for not telling his mother for 1 month. In other cases, children still question their decision to disclose, believing that they betrayed the perpetrators.

In the caretakers' group, the adults:

    a. Participate in the same activity as the children and share their own reactions to the disclosure.

    b. Are encouraged to empathize with their children's experience of isolation and fear that prolonged the silence. Caretakers also need to address feelings of resentment and disappointment with their children for not telling sooner.

    c. Those caretakers who had suspected or known of the molestation continue to explore their own fears that interfered with their being protective.

3. Letter to the Nonoffending Caretaker (Handouts 5-3 and 5-4)

In this activity, each child is asked to write a letter to the nonoffending parent/caretaker and share feelings about parental response to the disclosure of sexual abuse. The children are told that these letters are to be used to help express difficult feelings in group, and the letters may be shared with caretakers at the children's discretion. In this letter each child will address the possibility that the caretaker had knowledge of the abuse while it was occurring, will consider whether the caretaker believed the child, and will describe ways the caretaker could have been more supportive to the child.

Once the letters are written, the children take turns reading the letters out loud to the group. The letters are often self-effacing and apologetic. This continued self-blame and guilt can interfere with appropriately directed anger and works against healthy separation. The therapists must help the children to place some responsibility on the adults. The therapists must also normalize and permit feelings of anger, betrayal, and hurt, while acknowledging the discomfort that the children experience in admitting negative feelings about the important people upon whom they depend for nurturance and support.

In the caretakers' group, the adults:

    a. Write letters to their children in which they review their own reactions to learning about the molestation and consider ways they could have been more supportive. Many parents use this opportunity to apologize to their children for not being helpful or reassuring. Caretakers, who were not part of the child's life at the time of the disclosure, can use this letter to reinforce the child's decision to disclose and underscore their sense of responsibility for providing a safe home for the child.

    b. Are encouraged to share their letters with their children. This is an extremely important exercise because it facilitates communication between caretakers and children about the disclosure and, in many cases, the abuse itself. If time permits, and families are interested, the therapists should consider a mutual sharing of letters during a separate conjoint session for each individual family, to encourage further interaction and clarify and reinforce issues of adult responsibility. This is also an opportunity for caretakers who were molested as children to disclose their own victimization, in an effort to demonstrate understanding for their children's experience.

4. A Story about Court (Handout 5-5)

Following disclosure of sexual abuse, many children become involved in dependency, family, or criminal court. This is often a frightening experience and can further traumatize the children when it produces separations or when children are intimidated by perpetrators and their attorneys. This activity can be used with those group members who have already been to court, as well as with those who may be appearing shortly. This exercise allows children to gain some mastery by introducing them to the various court personnel and their roles.

Each child chooses a role and is given a brief written description of the character. Therapists may have to become involved in the selection process, as most of the children ask to play the "judge" so they can render the decision they had wished for in their own cases. Sometimes it works well to allow children to alternate roles during the role play. Once the roles are determined, the group members play out a courtroom scenario. The authors present a typical dependency court situation in Handout 5-5. Therapists can use the general structure to develop other scenarios that more closely describe the situations of the majority of children in any particular group. Children are encouraged to help each other to act out the parts.

Therapists use the group members' own court experiences to present strategies for court appearances, helping children to be assertive in this stressful situation and to identify whom they can ask for help when feeling pressured or confused. Group members seem to draw courage from hearing about the experiences of their peers in court. Children also express fears that offenders will retaliate following their testimony. One child countered every attempt at reassurance of his safety by group members and therapists, insisting that the perpetrator would summon superhuman strength to take immediate retribution upon him. His concern was greatly alleviated when he came to understand that his fear was partially a projection of his own rage and wish to retaliate.

In the caretakers' group, the adults:

    a. Develop strategies to support children through the trauma of court appearances.

    b. Explore the uncertainty about whether to allow their children to testify in criminal court when there is a possibility that the cases will be dismissed or the perpetrators will not be adequately punished.

    c. Prepare for the possibility that the court system may not validate their children's allegations.

TREATMENT CHALLENGES

    1. Caretakers may become so anxious about the content of their children's letters that they put pressure on the children to reveal the letters. Therapists should emphasize the importance of respecting the children's confidentiality and use this opportunity to explore the underlying anxiety and guilt.

2. Some caretakers may feel attacked by their children's expression of anger and disappointment, and may see the therapists as encouraging the children to blame the nonoffending caretakers for the abuse. Therapists should appreciate the feelings of guilt and failure that these adults are defending against, and help group members to distinguish between assessing responsibility and assigning blame.

3. Some caretakers continue to rationalize the offenders' behavior and present it to the children as somehow out of the offenders' control. This makes it very difficult for the children to feel justified in being angry and usually contributes to their silence. Therapists should explore what it would mean to the caretakers if the offenders were, in fact, in control of their abusive behavior.

4. Some children will no longer be living with the parents who heard the original disclosure, and writing a letter to an absent and rejecting parent may be quite painful. It is important to encourage these children to participate in this exercise and to reassure them that their new caretakers will also be writing letters to them in the adult group.

HANDOUT 5-1: KEEPING THE SECRET

ROLE PLAY #1

The Setting

Cathy and Jane were both molested by their soccer coach. One day after practice he asked Cathy and Jane to stay and watch videos; then he touched their private parts. Cathy didn't want to tell anyone because she was sure that she would be in trouble, everyone at school would find out, and her mom would make her give up soccer. Jane wanted to tell right away.

Questions

    a. How is Cathy feeling? How is Jane feeling?
    b. What will happen if the girls tell?
    c. What will happen if Jane tells and Cathy doesn't?
    d. If they tell, will they be believed?
    e. Whom can they tell?

Role Play

How can Jane help Cathy to tell what happened?

ROLE PLAY #2

The Setting

Joey was playing at a friend's house down the street when he decided to go home to get something. When he got to the front door it was locked. "That's funny," he thought, because he knew his sister, Susie, and his stepfather were at home. He went to the side of the house and peeked into his sister's room. He saw his sister lying on the bed crying. He also saw the back of his stepfather, who was putting on his pants.

Questions

    a. How did Joey feel about what he saw?
    b. What should he do now?
    c. Should he tell someone? Who can he tell?
    d. What would Susie want her brother to do?

Role Play

Joey tells Susie about what he saw.

ROLE PLAY #3

The Setting

Diane and Angela are in the same class. They have been best friends since kindergarten and have shared many secrets. Lately Angela has noticed that Diane is not acting like herself. She isn't as much fun as she used to be and always seems upset. One day Angela asked Diane if something was bothering her. Diane told Angela she would tell her only if she promised to keep it a secret. She warned Angela that if she ever told anyone their secret she would no longer be her friend and would tell all the other children in their class not to be friends with her. Angela promised to keep the secret and Diane then told her that her father has been touching her private parts.

Questions

    a. How does Diane feel?
    b. How does Angela feel?
    c. Should Angela keep the secret?
    d. Why do you think Diane told Angela?

Role Play

How can Angela help Diane tell someone?

ROLE PLAY #4

The Setting

Billy has been molested by his stepfather for the past 6 months. His stepfather owns several guns and takes Billy hunting sometimes. Billy's stepfather said that if he told anyone something awful would happen. Billy is really scared of his stepfather, but he has decided to tell his teacher about being molested anyway.

Questions

    a. How is Billy feeling?
    b. Do you think he has good reason to be afraid of his stepfather?
    c. Why has Billy decided now to tell his teacher?
    d. How could his teacher help Billy?

Role Play

Billy is trying to tell his teacher about what happened.

ROLE PLAY #5

The Setting

Bobby has been molested by his Uncle John for the past 3 years. Bobby always liked spending time with his uncle and still does except when he wants to touch Bobby's private parts. Bobby's dad died when he was a baby, and his uncle is sort of a second dad.

Questions

    a. Why is Bobby keeping this secret?
    b. What will happen if he tells?
    c. What does Bobby have to gain by telling?
       What does he have to lose?

Role Play

Bobby's mother wants him to spend the weekend with Uncle John. Bobby resists going in spite of his mother's insistence.

ROLE PLAY #6

The Setting

Frank has been molested by his older cousin Joe for a year. Joe told Frank that he would beat him up if Frank tells anyone that he was molested. Frank acts real tough with his friends but still does not tell anyone about Joe.

Questions

    a. Why hasn't Frank told anyone?
    b. Can anyone help Frank be safe from Joe?
    c. Why do you think Frank acts so tough with kids his own age?
    d. Why doesn't he tell one of his friends about being molested?

Role Play

Frank's mother brings him to a therapist because he fights so much with other kids.

Name _____

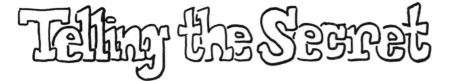

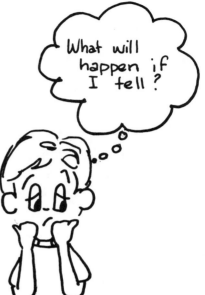

What will happen if I tell?

1. What did _____ tell you might happen if you told about being molested? _____
_____
_____

2. Describe how it felt to keep this secret. Did you want to tell someone? Who? _____
_____
_____
_____

3. Did you try to tell someone? How? _____
_____

4. How old were you when people found out you were being molested? _____

5. How did your parent(s) find out you were being molested? _____
_____

6. How did you feel after it was discovered? _____
_____

7. Did your parent believe you? If not, did this change? _____
_____

8. What happened after people knew? Who interviewed you? _____
_____

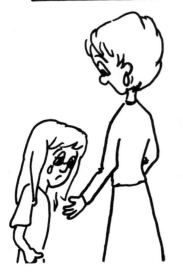

9. What happened to the perpetrator? Did you have to leave? _____
_____
_____
_____

10. Did the perpetrator admit or deny molesting you? What did the person say about it? _____
_____
_____
_____

HANDOUT 5-3: LETTER TO THE NON-OFFENDING CARETAKER

Date: _____

To: _____

When you found out about what was happening to me, I felt like

you _____

_____.

Some things that you said to me made me feel _____

_____ like when you told me _____

_____.

I have wanted to ask you if _____

_____

and _____.

I wish you would have _____

_____.

Some other things I want to tell you are _____

_____

_____

_____

_____

_____   _____

_____   _____

P.S. _____

HANDOUT 5-4: LETTER TO THE NON-OFFENDING CARETAKER

Date:_____

To:_____

When you found out about what was happening to me, I felt like you _____

_____

_____.

Some things that you said to me made me feel _____

_____ like when you told me _____

_____.

I have wanted to ask you if _____

_____

and _____.

I wish you would have _____

_____.

Some other things I want to tell you are _____

_____

_____

_____

_____

_____

_____

_____

_____   _____

                                                         _____

P.S. _____

HANDOUT 5-5: A STORY ABOUT COURT

THE SETTING

Jane is an 8-year-old girl who is living in a foster home. When she first told her mother that her stepfather had been molesting her, her mother did not believe her. Two months later there was a program on child abuse at school, and Jane told her teacher. The teacher was required to report the abuse, and a social worker went to speak with the mother. The mother told the worker that she couldn't believe that her husband would do such a thing, and so the worker took Jane to a foster home for her safety. This is the first court hearing to decide if Jane can come home. The mother, who is still not certain whether to believe Jane, did have the stepfather move out. The judge must decide if the mother can protect Jane from more abuse.

Jane

Jane is very upset. She does not like being in a foster home and away from her family; she wants to go home. She feels responsible for her stepfather having to move out, and she fears that both of her parents are very mad at her. She wonders whether the molestation is her fault and blames herself for letting it go on, but she remembers how scared she felt, hoping that her stepfather would stop touching her and that her family would go back to the way they used to be before. She believes that if she tells everyone that she made up the whole thing, she can go home. But, if she returns home and her stepfather is also allowed to return home, she worries he will try to molest her again or worse.

Jane's Lawyer

A lawyer is assigned to Jane by the judge to protect her and to make certain that she will be safe. The lawyer can help Jane to tell the judge about the abuse. Jane and her lawyer must meet together before going to court, because the lawyer needs to know exactly what happened in order to help Jane get ready to testify in court.

Mother

Jane's mother is also very upset. She doesn't know whom to believe. Her daughter said that her stepfather molested her, but the stepfather denies the whole thing. Jane has made up many stories before, so it's very hard to know if this is a story too. The mother wants Jane to come home but doesn't want to lose her husband. She doesn't want to think that her husband could do such a thing, but at times she feels sad for her daughter and mad at her husband, believing that he probably did molest Jane. The mother is also mad at herself for not having protected Jane from being molested. She feels guilty and wonders if she really is a good mother.

Stepfather

The stepfather knows he could be in a lot of trouble. He did molest his stepdaughter, but he never thought she would tell. Jane has made up stories before, so he thinks that if he just keeps saying he didn't do anything, he will eventually be able to go home. He is worried, however, about the interview he had with the therapist—he's not sure if he's convinced her. He is also afraid he will lose his wife and go to jail. But, sometimes, late at night, he feels badly for his stepdaughter and wonders why he molested her.

Mother and Stepfather's Lawyer

The lawyer for the parents is responsible for being sure that they are protected. The lawyer will try to make the judge think that this is another one of Jane's stories. The lawyer will try to make the stepfather seem like a good person who should be able to come home to his family and will show the mother as being very concerned about Jane.

Therapist

Jane has had four visits with the therapist. Now the judge is asking the therapist to say if she believes that Jane was molested. Jane says she made up the story, but the therapist believes the molestation did happen, because children usually do not make up stories about being molested and they often worry about anger from their parents. The therapist is only willing to recommend that Jane go home to her mother if the stepfather remains out of the home and all family members are in therapy.

Social Worker

The social worker is ordered by the judge to meet all the members of the family and to tell the judge whether it is safe for Jane to return home. To make this decision, the social worker will need to ask everyone in the family many questions about how Jane will be protected.

Judge

The judge is in charge of the court. The judge hears all the facts, which include written reports and testimony by different witnesses, such as Jane, her mother, and the therapist. The judge then considers all the information and makes a decision in the best interests of the child. The judge may also ask questions in order to better understand what is being said. The judge may decide to talk with Jane alone, especially if Jane is uncomfortable.

Other Courtroom People

There are three other important people in all courtrooms who assist the judge. These roles can be used when additional parts are needed.

1. The bailiff—keeps order in the court and calls each person to testify.
2. The court clerk—gives the oath (a promise to tell the truth) to each witness.
3. The court reporter—records every word said during the hearing or trial.

ROLE PLAY

How do Jane, her mother and stepfather, the lawyers, and everybody else act in court? What does the judge decide?

MODULE 6 My Family

PURPOSE

Once the initial trauma of disclosure has subsided, child victims often remain preoccupied with whether they "did the right thing" by telling about the abuse. The children often feel a sense of responsibility for the major lifestyle changes that inevitably occur in these families. In some cases, past child–parent problems contribute to family dysfunction, and children continue to show excessive concern for their parents' needs at the expense of their own.

In addition, victims must often give up familiar social and family supports. In an incest situation, children who remain at home may have to accept a lower standard of living and less time with a single parent who must now provide financially for the family. The parent may also begin to pursue new social interests or to spend time with the perpetrator away from home. There is an increase in conflict among siblings as they wrestle with feelings of responsibility for the loss of the perpetrator and anger at each other for their perceived roles in the sexual abuse. Furthermore, family members remain in a state of perpetual anxiety about court-ordered visits with perpetrators. Victims feel pressured to comply with the wishes of siblings and caretakers. Children who want to maintain contact with an absent parent may feel compelled to complain about the visits to please an angry caretaker. Children who prefer to avoid the perpetrator may deny any negative feelings because they believe that the nonoffending caretaker plans reunification and that their sisters and brothers miss the absent parent. Still other victims' worries and fears about anticipated visits are exacerbated by continual expressions of anger and dread by the caretakers.

Following extrafamilial abuse, parents may become increasingly protective and attempt to keep the victim "in sight" at all times. They no longer believe in their own or their child's ability to judge the trustworthiness of other adults.

In still other cases, the child is placed out of the home, either in the foster care system or with relatives who may be critical of the parents. The child must then learn to adjust to a new family and to the uncertainty about visitation or eventual return to natural parents. The new caretakers may be ill prepared to understand and manage long-standing behavioral problems or expected difficulties in adjustment. The purpose of this module is to facilitate more honest and effective communication within the family unit.

113

OBJECTIVES

1. Decrease feelings of responsibility for losses in the family.
2. Help children and caretakers to anticipate the effects of changes within the family and develop coping skills.
3. Reinforce the role of the caretakers in their families and give children permission to relinquish their parenting function.
4. Assist children and caretakers to prepare for visitations with alleged or convicted perpetrators.
5. Reduce the children's anxiety about asking for parental permission to become increasingly involved in activities and relationships outside of the home.
6. Prepare caretakers for their children's inevitable need to look beyond the family for interest and enjoyment.

THERAPEUTIC CONSIDERATIONS

To facilitate families adjustment to changes in roles and relationships, therapists should:

1. Appreciate the variety of living situations represented in each group.
2. Predict that caretakers are bound to experience increased discomfort at the possibility of their children's seeking more independence.
3. Understand that many children who felt unprotected in the past will resist opportunities to individuate.
4. Respect the children's need to idealize their living situation and recognize that there may be increased disruptiveness or defiance in group as anger is displaced onto the therapists.
5. Accept that children who have been placed outside the home may defend against fears of further abandonment by alienating individual group members or devaluing the group experience.
6. Reinforce efforts by newly single parents to develop assertiveness and to "take charge" within their families.
7. Anticipate the conflict among various adult group members who need to defend their personal positions about reuniting with or separating from the perpetrators.
8. Recognize that the adults may become resistant when encouraged to examine how they may be contributing to their children's discomfort about visitations with perpetrators.
9. Expect that some caretakers who are court-ordered to treatment may externalize blame for difficulties within their families.

ACTIVITIES FOR MODULE #6 (2–3 sessions)

1. My New Family

In this exercise, each child is given a large piece of paper and is asked to draw a line down the middle of the page. On one side, the child draws a picture of his/her family before the disclosure; on the other half, the child draws a picture of the family now. For each picture, the child is asked to portray a typical day at home with the family members. Once the pictures are completed, therapists then help the children to examine how their families have changed, including relationships with siblings, and how responsibilities in the families may have been altered. In one group, a child drew identical pictures on both sides of the page with her father prominently placed in the center. This girl was then able to express her discomfort with her mother's continuing involvement with the perpetrator.

In the caretakers' group, the adults explore:

   a. The ways their children have been affected by the family changes, including relationships with siblings and other relatives.
   b. The most significant changes they have experienced personally since the disclosure by their children.
   c. The expectations they have for their children about family responsibilities.
   d. How their relationships with their children have changed since the disclosure.

2. Parents (Handout 6-1)

In this activity, the children complete a checklist that focuses more directly on how the children feel about their parents and how they believe their parents feel about them. The therapists then use the answers to help the children explore these feelings and to encourage the children to communicate concerns, fears, and wishes directly. Children who are not living with their parents can still use this activity to explore relationships in their current home. Children often mark "yes" to the statement "My parent(s) want me to be perfect," acknowledging strong feelings of responsibility to meet unrealistic parental expectations.

In the caretakers' group, the adults:

   a. Consider how they believe their children feel about them.
   b. Address ways they can encourage their children to share concerns and feelings about the family.
   c. Explore their own feelings about their families and changes they would like to make.
   d. Determine ways they can influence changes in their families.

3. Sisters and Brothers (Handout 6-2)

In this exercise, the victims complete a checklist which examines how they perceive the reactions of their siblings following disclosure of the molestation. A space is also provided to write down additional thoughts or feelings the children would like to share with their sisters and brothers. The therapists can use the written responses to help the children to address issues of guilt, self-blame, anger, and confusion that often occur among siblings, especially when the disclosure directly affects the siblings' relationship with the perpetrators or when siblings witnessed or had knowledge of the abuse prior to disclosure. In many cases, children report that they feel obligated to endure monitored visits with the perpetrators because of their siblings. Others voice anger at siblings who disclosed "without their permission."

In the caretakers' group, the adults:

a. Consider the special needs of sisters and brothers when the focus of concern and attention is on the victims.
b. Address their own concerns about how to balance protection of the victims with the desire of siblings to remain involved with the perpetrators, recognizing that siblings may also be at risk.
c. Examine the possible impact on their families when siblings have not been told about the molestation.

4. Visiting the Perpetrator (Handout 6-3)

In this activity, the children are given an opportunity to examine their many conflicting feelings about spending time with the person who molested them. As with past role plays, several common scenarios are represented and again the stories can be altered to better correlate with the needs of the children in a particular group. Following the role plays, the group members often express a variety of concerns about visits. One girl stated she did not want to see her father until he "apologized and got into counseling." Another boy wanted to visit his father so he would not feel "left out" when his siblings went on monitored outings. Still other children complain that perpetrators pressure them verbally or continue to treat them in inappropriate ways even in front of monitors. Therapists must explore these allegations carefully and consider reporting them to children's services or the court. Therapists can use this exercise to not only validate the children's struggles but to assist them in preparing for and surviving visits to decrease continued feelings of victimization.

In the caretakers' group, the adults:

a. Practice the same role plays in Handout 6-3 to increase their capacity to understand the various conflicts that occur when visitations with perpetrators are required.
b. Explore their own feelings/fears about the visitations and the monitors, and consider how these reactions may influence their children's experiences.
c. Acknowledge their own helplessness and how it inhibits their ability to prepare the children to cope with visits.
d. Develop ways to provide support for their children and lessen children's feelings of guilt and responsibility for caretakers.

5. Asking Permission (Handout 6-4)

The therapists provide situations in which children must gain permission from their caretakers to increase time spent outside of their families. The children first consider their own feelings about being away from home and possible reactions by their caretakers to each request. Then, in front of the group, the children practice asking for permission, with one group member taking the role of the child and one group member playing the adult. Each child should have the opportunity to take the role of caretaker. The therapists may even want to consider the possibility of combining the children's and the caretakers' groups for this exercise. During one session, the "mothers" were all very strict and refused to allow their daughters out of the house under any circumstances because of possible risk of abuse. In another group, the role plays led to a fruitful examination of how children "get their way" with adults.

In the caretakers' group, the adults:

a. Evaluate their feelings about their children's need to move apart from them.
b. Review the children's exercise and consider how they might respond to each of the requests by their children.
c. Address concerns about their children's ability to be self-protective and fears that their children might victimize others.
d. Practice the "Role Plays for Caretakers" (Handout 6-5) to increase empathy for their children and develop tools to improve communication at home.

TREATMENT CHALLENGES

1. As evidenced in various ways throughout the group experience, the therapists may again be viewed as either encouraging insubordination by the children or causing a split between the children and their caretakers. Therapists should encourage the adults to explore their feelings about separation and loss, and begin to educate them about age-appropriate attempts at independence.

2. New caretakers who do not take responsibility for any of the victims' difficulties may insist that they "know how" to talk to their children and do not need to "practice" effective communication. Therapists may want to suggest that these caretakers share their knowledge and experience with the group; this may reduce their need to devalue other group members.

3. Some caretakers, who are considering reunification with the perpetrators, may begin to withdraw from active participation in the group if they feel criticized by other caretakers. It is important for the therapists to help group members identify common concerns about the children, and at the same time to support different viewpoints. For example, it may be possible for a parent to provide adequate protection for a child and still consider a relationship in the future with the perpetrator.

4. Some children will react to talking about their families with expressions of boredom: "Do we have to do another handout/role play?" Therapists should be aware of the defensive nature of these complaints and acknowledge possible discomfort with the issues addressed in this module.

5. Many caretakers will again use the group to express feelings of persecution from the legal system, claiming that "my family would be just fine" if social services would "leave us alone." Therapists must acknowledge the reality of the current legal situation for some families and then shift the focus to areas in which caretakers can experience some control, such as setting effective limits or providing emotional support for their children.

Name: _____

Parents

My parent(s):	YES	NO	SOMETIMES
1. would like it if I studied harder.	——	——	——
2. want me to be happy.	——	——	——
3. need my help a lot.	——	——	——
4. understand my feelings.	——	——	——
5. think I'm a great kid.	——	——	——
6. are always too busy.	——	——	——
7. are too strict.	——	——	——
8. are not fair.	——	——	——
9. are often tired and unhappy.	——	——	——
10. know when I am worried.	——	——	——
11. want me to be perfect.	——	——	——
12. always want to know what I'm doing.	——	——	——
13. treat me differently.	——	——	——
14. make me feel safe.	——	——	——
15. give me too many chores.	——	——	——

Name: _____

Sisters and Brothers

	YES	NO	I DON'T KNOW
My sisters and brothers:			
1. knew I was being molested.	___	___	___
2. told someone I was being molested.	___	___	___
3. don't know I was being molested.	___	___	___
4. blame me for what happened.	___	___	___
5. feel sorry for me because I was molested.	___	___	___
6. think I get treated special.	___	___	___
7. are mad that they can't be with _____.	___	___	___
8. can't understand why everyone makes such a fuss over me.	___	___	___
9. worry about me.	___	___	___
10. get treated better than I do.	___	___	___

I wish I could tell my sister or brother_____

_____

_____

_____

_____

I wish my sister or brother would _____

_____

_____

_____

_____

HANDOUT 6-3: VISITING THE PERPETRATOR

ROLE PLAY #1

Karen is feeling very confused. The judge has said that she is supposed to spend 2 hours every Sunday with her father as long as her aunt is with them. She misses her father very much and is sad that he moved out of the house, even though she is glad that he is no longer molesting her. She gets really excited as it gets closer to the weekend but she has to pretend she doesn't want to go. Her mother says mean things about her father and wants him to go away and leave the family alone. Whenever Karen says something nice about her father, her mother says "How can you still love someone who molested you?"

Questions

    a. How does Karen feel when she pretends she doesn't want to go with her father?
    b. Is it sometimes hard for Karen to have fun on her visits with father? Why?
    c. Is it O.K. for Karen to want to be with her father?

Role Play

Karen tries to tell her mother how she really feels about being with her father.

ROLE PLAY #2

The Setting

Ruth feels embarrassed and humiliated that her stepfather, John, molested her and is also very scared that he will try to touch her again or get even with her for telling on him. John went to jail for 6 months and will be getting out very soon. Ruth knows that her mom still loves John and wants to be with him as soon as the judge will let John come back home. The judge has already said that John can be with the family every Sunday with mom as the monitor. Ruth is mad and hurt that her mother wants John back and doesn't believe that mom can really keep her safe. On the other hand, she feels guilty for hurting mom and doesn't want mom to stop loving her. Ruth also knows that her 3-year-old sister wants "her daddy."

Questions

    a. Is Ruth going to be safe during the visits with John? Why? Why not?
    b. Why does mom want John back?
    c. Does Ruth think that her mom loves her?

Role Play

Ruth tries to tell her mom how she feels about the visits and her fears that John may try to molest her again.

ROLE PLAY #3

The Setting

Gary and Steven are very frightened of their father, who sexually molested them and hit them many times and also beat up their mother. Father denied that he ever hurt anyone and the judge believed him. Father and mother are now divorced but father is allowed to have his sons spend all day Saturday with him at his parents' house where he now lives. The court did agree that for now the grandparents could be the monitors. Gary and Steven don't think that their grandparents will protect them and are scared every minute that something "bad will happen." Several days before each visit, the boys feel sick and want to stay home from school; after the visits they often fight a lot with each other. Their mother is depressed and fearful and can't make Gary or Steven feel better.

Questions

    a. Why do the boys fight with each other after they visit their father?
    b. What do Gary and Steven want their mother to do?
    c. How do the boys feel about the judge's decision?
    d. How do the boys feel now about telling the secret?
    e. How can mother help the boys to cope with the visits?

Role Play

The boys ask their mother to help them figure out ways to feel safe on the visits with their father.

Asking Permission

ROLE PLAYS

In each role play, the child asks the caretaker for permission to:

1. visit a friend's house after school.
2. go to a school dance at night.
3. go to the movies with a group of boys and girls.
4. take the bus to the shopping mall.
5. spend the night at a friend's house.
6. go to overnight summer camp for a week.
7. go on vacation with a new friend's family.
8. spend the night with the rest of the team at the coach's house.

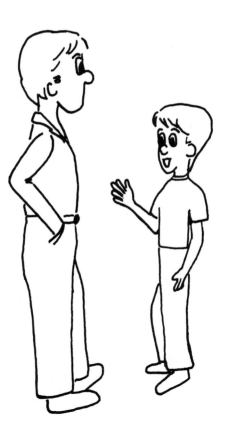
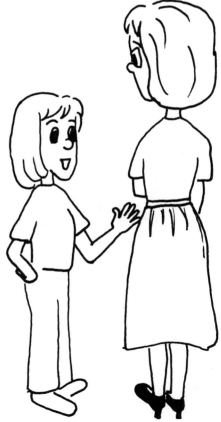

HANDOUT 6-5: ROLE PLAYS FOR CARETAKERS

ROLE PLAY #1

Sally is 13 years old and is in the seventh grade. This is the third school in 3 years for Sally, and she very much wants to make friends. This has been very difficult for her, because she believes that being molested makes her different somehow and that others don't like her. A 14-year-old boy named Brian in the eighth grade has just invited Sally on a group date to the movies and out for pizza. Brian is a boy in one of her classes with whom she has become friendly, and she likes him. She needs to give Brian her answer by tomorrow and will have to ask her mother tonight. She is nervous about this.

Sally's mother has been feeling somewhat guilty about all the moves the family has made, and worries about Sally not having any friends. She also worries about how she will react when Sally shows an interest in boys and dating. Sally was molested by her stepfather, and the mother still wonders how that may have effected Sally's judgment and ability to protect herself. Sally and her mother have not talked about the abuse since it was disclosed 3 years ago, and in fact their relationship has become stormy. The mother wonders if she has become overprotective of her daughter. On the other hand, she knows that young teenagers are often impulsive, and she wants to be certain that she provides adequate protection and concern.

Role Play

When her mother gets home from work, Sally is going to ask for permission to accept the date with Brian.

ROLE PLAY #2

Mom works full-time to support the family. She cannot afford child care, and she must ask her oldest daughter Cynthia (age 10) to watch the two younger children after school. Mom feels somewhat guilty about this, because she knows Cynthia needs to be with children her own age and Cynthia has been wanting to join some after-school activities. This babysitting arrangement seems to be working out well, but Mom has recently noticed that Cynthia has not been doing her chores around the house. This has made more work for Mom and there have been many arguments. Also, Cynthia has been looking somewhat unkempt, showering less often, and dressing sloppily. Mom feels overwhelmed. She feels she is doing the best she can, and needs Cynthia to cooperate and take charge when she isn't home.

Cynthia is unhappy. On the one hand, she resents having to watch her younger sisters and not having time for herself. On the other hand, she is the oldest and feels a sense of responsibility to help the family. She also worries about Mom, who has been looking very tired lately. She knows Mom is angry with her for not doing the chores, but she hasn't felt like it. Also, she has been tired and irritable, and feels less interested in her appearance. She would like to talk to Mom about how she is feeling, but fears that either Mom will get angry or she will worry Mom.

Role Play

When she gets home from work, Mom plans to talk to Cynthia about her behavior.

MODULE 7 Taking Care of Myself

PURPOSE

For children who have been sexually misused, feelings of shame, worthlessness, and helplessness are incorporated into their self-concept, and they do not view themselves as having the power to influence the events in their lives. This attitude is often reinforced by caretakers and may be especially unacceptable to boys, who believe they should have been able to defend themselves in spite of intimidation or force by the perpetrators. The pervasive sense of badness and vulnerability often places these children at risk for further sexual molestation. On the other hand, in an effort to overcome these feelings of inadequacy and to increase mastery and control, these children often touch their peers or adults without permission, and may attempt to recreate the abuse experience through the sexual victimization of others. Finally, an overall lack of confidence obscures the children's ability to see either themselves or others realistically, thereby interfering with the give-and-take of mutually satisfying friendships.

It seems advisable to place special emphasis on these issues at a stage in treatment when the children have addressed many of the feelings associated with being molested and may be more receptive to a constructive self-appraisal. Up to now, the group has provided an opportunity to test out and subsequently minimize fears of being different and expectations of being ridiculed and rejected. In addition, therapeutic limit setting has reinforced the idea that the children are entitled to protection and must learn to respect the rights of others. At this point in the group process, the children have developed a strong cohesive unit based on the sharing of very personal experiences, and there is increased interest in the evaluation of interpersonal communications. This module aims to enhance the self-esteem that has begun to re-emerge through the validation and normalization processes initiated during the first part of the program. The therapists must also help the children and the caretakers to develop the tools to determine who can provide emotional support and what steps are necessary to negotiate threatening situations. Latency-age children must attain a positive self-image, respect boundaries, and develop the ability to be assertive in order to enjoy healthy peer relationships.

OBJECTIVES

1. Assist children and caretakers to identify and appreciate their strengths and to confirm that they are capable of making self-protective decisions.

129

2. Help group members to recognize potentially dangerous situations.
3. Reinforce the importance of respecting the right of others to a personal space.
4. Give children permission to be assertive and to say "No!"
5. Reinforce a sense of being "in charge," thereby decreasing the need to dominate others.
6. Discourage the victim role by helping children to develop effective ways of taking care of their own needs.
7. Improve social skills by encouraging children to practice providing positive and negative feedback in ways that decrease defensiveness and demonstrate caring.
8. Clarify misconceptions about appropriate and inappropriate touching.

THERAPEUTIC CONSIDERATIONS

To help group members to attain a sense of mastery, therapists should:

1. Recognize that children who feel undeserving of friends may adopt the attributes of more dominant group members, decreasing their capacity to become assertive in their own right.
2. Accept that they themselves may be frustrated in their efforts to encourage group members to confront each other.
3. Anticipate that children and caretakers may view their efforts as useless and ineffective when their requests of other group members are ignored.
4. Respect that there may be cultural or religious differences regarding the acceptability of assertive behavior, and understand that in some families children are discouraged from challenging adults.
5. Recognize that some parents, who were unable to be assertive with the perpetrators, will again experience feelings of guilt, helplessness, and anger.
6. Acknowledge that some children view compliments as manipulative and requiring something in return, as in their molestation experience. Feelings of guilt may resurface as they are reminded of their past relationships with the perpetrators.
7. Appreciate that there are certain circumstances where it might be better for children to avoid confrontation, and help them to learn to differentiate.
8. Help the children to achieve a balance between an acceptance of feelings of helplessness and empowerment to act assertively in threatening situations.
9. Expect that when group members begin to address inappropriate attempts to master feelings of helplessness, there may be disclosures that some group members have themselves been engaged in sexual activity with other children. This can result in great anxiety among others in group and can lead to scapegoating. On the other hand, these admissions provide an opportunity for therapists to help children differentiate between innocent sexual curiosity and coercive, unacceptable, and abusive behavior.

ACTIVITIES FOR MODULE #7 (4–6 sessions)

1. Nice Things About . . . (Handout 7-1)

In this exercise, the children have an opportunity to give and to receive positive feedback. Each child writes down two nice things on separate activity sheets for each group member and each therapist. The therapists also write down "nice things about" each group member, focusing their comments on the children's participation in group, such as "You are willing to share your feelings in group." The therapists then collect and distribute the compliments to each child. The children and the therapists take turns reading out loud all of the nice feedback they have received, and children are encouraged to take home their compliments and share them with caretakers. This is usually a very positive experience for the children, who receive confirmation that they are liked by others.

In the caretakers' group, the adults:

    a. Participate in the same exercise as the children, which reinforces the importance of receiving positive feedback as adults.

    b. Consider the impact of positive reinforcement on self-esteem.

    c. Review the ways they were given positive messages as children and how they are praised as adults.

    d. Learn more effective ways to praise their children.

2. How I See Myself

In this exercise, the children each make a collage by selecting magazine pictures that represent how they see themselves. Each child shows his/her collage to the group, and the other group members consider whether they view the presenter in the same way. The therapists help the children to examine their view of themselves and how this is influenced by their caretakers. One girl chose several pictures of obese people because she claimed she was "fat." When other girls expressed confusion because they did not think she was overweight, she revealed that her mother always complained that she "eats too much." Although this exercise comes in the second half of the group, it can be useful to present it in one of the beginning modules and then reintroduce it later, to compare changes in appraisals of self-worth as treatment progresses.

In the caretakers' group, the adults consider:

    a. How they believe their children view themselves.

    b. The qualities they value most in their children and how these are communicated.

    c. The qualities they value most in themselves.

    d. Their memories about the positive and negative messages they received when they were children, and the impact of these on their capacity to praise their own children.

3. Taking Care of Yourself

The therapists show the children one of the many available videos that demonstrate the basic ways to anticipate, avoid, or cope with potentially dangerous situations. It is most helpful to use a film that presents a variety of vignettes in which children react to different threatening situations. The group members can consider the feelings of the children in the stories, and identify similar experiences they have encountered. Then, using the same vignettes in the film or additional ones provided by the therapists, the children role-play scenarios in which they are at risk for potential abuse. The children practice refusals, explore options for getting away, and consider whom they can tell. Each child should have the opportunity to play both the potential victim and the perpetrator. The role plays are important, because as one boy stated, "It's easy to plan what to do," but he might be "too scared in the real situation."

In the caretakers' group, the adults:

    a. Examine how they prepare children to be cautious and self-protective.
    b. Decide on the necessary information that all children must have to cope with unfamiliar or scary situations that might occur.
    c. Watch the same film as the children's group and consider how their children would have coped with the different scenarios. It is often productive to combine the children and the caretakers for this exercise, and focus on family rules for self-protective behavior, encouraging caretakers to reinforce their children's efforts at assertiveness.

4. Different Touches (Handout 7-2)

Although learning about different touches is often focused on younger children, latency-age children continue to have difficulty discriminating the finer distinctions. For example, an injection by the doctor may be considered a touch that "feels bad," but it is not abusive; or an innocent hug by a mother for her son may be appropriate and feel good, but may also be sexually arousing to the boy, causing confusion and guilt. More overtly, some children will engage in sexualized play, not realizing that this behavior may be inappropriate or abusive. This exercise explores these ambiguous situations, which are often unclear and may provoke anxiety.

The children complete a checklist in which they consider what touches "feel good" or "feel bad" to them. In some cases, the children may not know how they feel about certain touches. There is also space available for children to give their own examples of touches that they like or do not like. The therapists help the group members to explore their ambivalence, to differentiate between uncomfortable and/or potentially abusive touches, and to consider how children can decide whether a particular touch is acceptable. This is a complex exercise because of the numerous variables that determine whether or not a touch is appropriate, including persistent confusion about what it means to be molested or to "molest someone".

Many children and their caretakers remain unclear about the definition of molestation and confused about what behaviors are unacceptable. For example, one mother denied her own victimization as a child because she never had intercourse with her step-father. Some children generalize molestation to other aggressive behaviors; one girl thought she had molested a peer because she hit the child. These responses allow therapists the opportunity to review and clarify the meaning of sexual molestation. When appropriate, this exercise can be expanded from discussion of general issues about touching to a more specific focus on when sexual activity is acceptable and when it is abusive. Although some past sexual experimentation may be expected, therapists must intervene with those children who admit perpetration of others with additional individual or group treatment.

Finally, the therapists review ways that the children can avoid or stop touches that seem inappropriate or make them feel uncomfortable or scared. When a child acknowledges discomfort with physical affection by caretakers, it may be helpful to address this in a conjoint session where the therapist can clarify the feelings and provide support for the child and the adult.

In the caretakers' group, the adults:

   a. Discuss how they teach their children about good and bad touches.
   b. Explore possible ways they may have pressured their children to tolerate nonabusive but uncomfortable touches, (e.g., hugs from relatives).
   c. Consider how they might respond if their children rejected or withdrew from their own demonstrations of physical affection.
   d. Recognize how their own misunderstanding about the molestation may affect their ability to stop inappropriate sexual activities of their children with peers or siblings.

5. Being Assertive (Handout 7-3)

This activity introduces the notion that each child has the right to expect fair treatment from others. The therapists tell the children that when a friend says or does something that makes them uncomfortable, they should tell that person how they feel and what they want. This exercise provides the children with the opportunity and the tools to be assertive with peers in a way that does not devalue or hurt others. Of course this first requires a discussion about criticism, including how it feels to be criticized (e.g., hurt, angry, rejected) and common reactions to criticism (e.g., talk back, withdraw, cry, ignore it). The group members then participate in role plays in which one child is uncomfortable or upset with a friend's behavior. For each circumstance, the child considers the feelings engendered by the friend's behavior, the possible risks of confronting that friend, and how the friend may feel when confronted. The child then practices the confrontation. Each group member should have the opportunity to play both parts.

As with other role plays, it is helpful to have the therapists play out the first scenario, reinforcing the importance of focusing on the behavior and not attacking a person's general character (e.g., "I wish you would stop telling me what to do" instead of "You are so bossy"). Children can be helped to state the behavior that upsets them, express how the behavior makes them feel, and make a request for change. It is also important for therapists to help the children to consider times when it might be best to avoid confrontation. In one group, a child was being repeatedly tormented by another group member who alternated between befriending and rejecting the child. Although other group members noticed and commented often on the abusive behavior, the child admitted she "put up with" the girl because she was "her only friend." This exercise encouraged her to take the risk and inform the girl that she would no longer "let her be mean" and that the abusive girl would "have to decide" about their friendship.

In the caretakers' group, the adults consider:

a. How their children respond to confrontation and criticism.
b. How they themselves respond to confrontation and criticism.
c. How they encourage or discourage their children to stand up for their rights.
d. Their own history of assertiveness and how this might affect their children.
e. How they can be more appropriately assertive in setting limits for their children.

ADDITIONAL RESOURCES

There are many excellent videotapes and activities that address issues of self-esteem and assertiveness. Some resources that the authors have used often in group are:

1. *Better safe than sorry II* [Videotape]. (Available from Film Fair Communication [Distributor], 10900 Ventura Blvd., P.O. Box 728, Studio City, CA, 91604)
   This video presents a variety of potentially dangerous situations that may confront children and provides techniques for self-protection.
2. *Better safe than sorry II* (2nd ed.) [Videotape]. (Available from Film Fair Communication [Distributor], 10900 Ventura Blvd., P.O. Box 728, Studio City, CA, 91604)
   This version uses latency-age children to present the vignettes and the important material to be learned.
3. *Strong kids, safe kids* [Video cassette]. (Available at most videocassette retail outlets or from Paramount Pictures, 5555 Melrose Ave., Hollywood, CA 90038)
4. Beck, T. G. (1984). *The talking and telling about touching game.* (Available from Victim Assistance Program, P.O. Box 444, Akron, OH 44309)
   This activity focuses on the importance of self-protectiveness and disclosure.
5. MacFarlane, K., & Cunningham, C. (1988). *Steps to healthy touching.* FL: Kidsrights.

This book addresses the problem of children who abuse other children, and contains a wide array of activities that promote self-esteem and healthy assertiveness.

6. Palmer, P. (1977). *Liking myself*. San Luis Obispo, CA: Impact.
    This book provides many activities related to self-esteem.

7. Palmer, P. (1977). *The mouse, the monster and me*. San Luis Obispo, CA: Impact.
    This book deals primarily with assertiveness.

TREATMENT CHALLENGES

1. Caretakers may again become concerned that therapists are encouraging defiance by permitting children to be assertive. Therapists must explore the adults' understanding about what it means to be assertive and clarify how assertiveness differs from aggressiveness. Therapists can also reinforce the positive aspects of children' experiencing some mastery over their relationships with others, which may reduce the risk of further victimization, while at the same time supporting the caretakers in the parenting role.

2. Some caretakers may charge that the therapists are discouraging their children from being physically affectionate with them. Therapists should recognize that these complaints are usually related to the separation concerns that have already emerged in regard to various other exercises. In addition, caretakers must be reminded that children who have been touched inappropriately are often distrustful of physical closeness, and that this distrust should not be confused with the withdrawal of affection.

3. In some cases, children will be unable to tolerate any critical discussion of their behavior, resulting in withdrawal or defensive attacks on others. Other children may use this opportunity to scapegoat disruptive or inattentive group members, further alienating them from the group. Therapists must set limits against attacks on others and must provide additional support for group members who are confronted, focusing exclusively on the specific behavior and not allowing character assassinations.

4. Children and adults may openly complain about a certain group member when that member is not present, but say nothing when the member returns to group. Therapists should help group members to explore their discomfort with direct confrontation. If appropriate, therapists can allow the group members to practice what they would like to tell the absent member when he/she returns. In some cases, the group may want to select a spokesperson (usually one of the therapists) to introduce the subject.

5. As cohesion and trust develop, some group members may spontaneously reveal that they have "molested" others. However, therapists must be aware that children who have been involved in sex play are often

unwilling to move beyond a superficial accounting of the behavior. While this does provide initial relief, further exploration is critical in order to reduce the children's sense of shame and the likelihood that they will again act out sexually. Unfortunately, therapists' attempts to address this issue are often resisted and perceived as condemnation. In addition, children who have not perpetrated become extremely anxious and often disrupt the group discussion. Efforts to respond to these disclosures by introducing additional structured activities in group are usually unsuccessful. Children who molest are probably best served with individual treatment or a group designed specifically for abuse reactive victims. Therapists may want to utilize the workbook "Steps To Healthy Touching" listed in the Additional Resources when treating child per- petrators.

Nice things about _____
   1. _____

      _____

   2. _____

      _____

- -

Nice things about _____
   1. _____

      _____

   2. _____

      _____

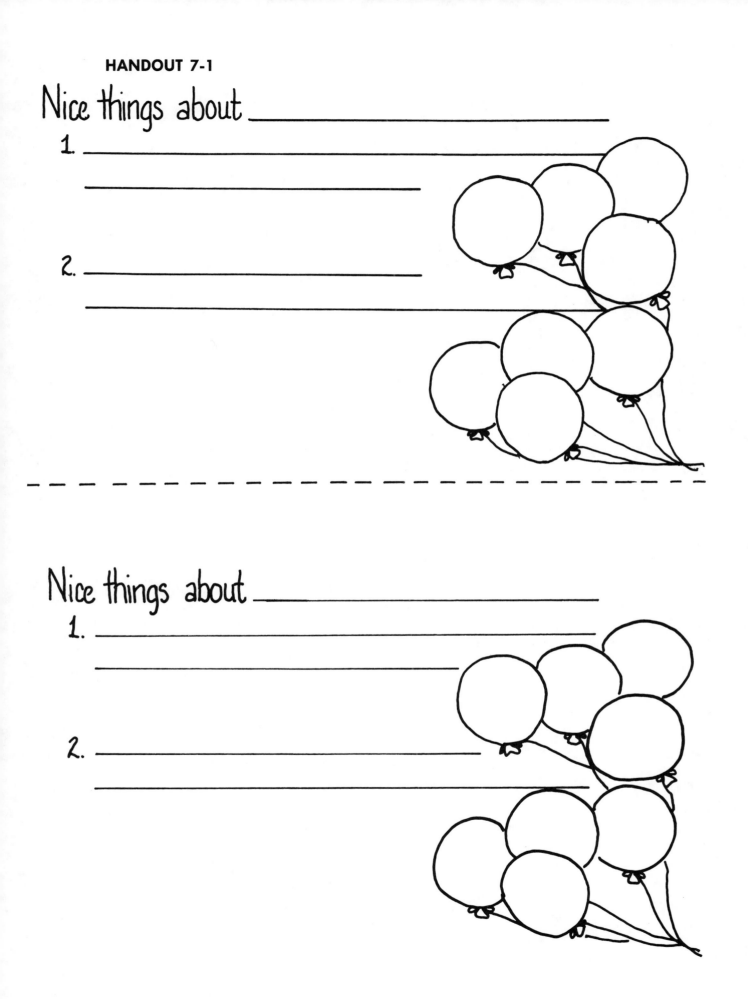

Name _____

Different Touches

	FEELS GOOD	I DON'T KNOW	FEELS BAD
1. A classmate pushes you while you're in line for lunch.	____	____	____
2. Your favorite uncle always wants to wrestle with you, sometimes when you don't want to play.	____	____	____
3. Your friend's father hugs you goodbye.	____	____	____
4. You get hit by a baseball by accident.	____	____	____
5. The babysitter always wants to help you take a bath.	____	____	____
6. Your doctor gives you a shot.	____	____	____
7. Your softball coach tells you that you've done a good job and gives you a pat on the rear.	____	____	____
8. _____ _____	____	____	____
9. _____ _____	____	____	____
10. _____ _____	____	____	____

Being Assertive
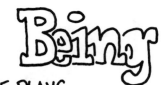
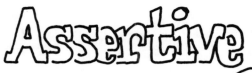

ROLE PLAYS

What would you do if :

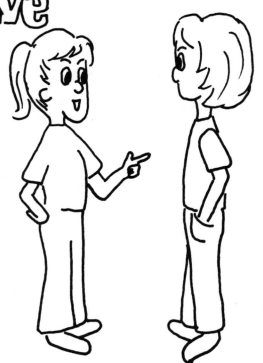

1. You are sitting with a friend at lunch and another child comes over and joins you. Suddenly the new child and your friend begin whispering and you are left out.

2. You find out that a classmate you like has not invited you to his/her birthday party.

3. Your friend borrows your _____ and doesn't return it.

4. You tell your friend a secret and find out that she/he has told other kids.

5. Another group member is always interrupting and acting silly when you try to talk.

6. A child you don't know moves ahead of you in the lunch line.

7. On your way to school, a bigger kid tells you to give him your lunch money or he'll beat you up.

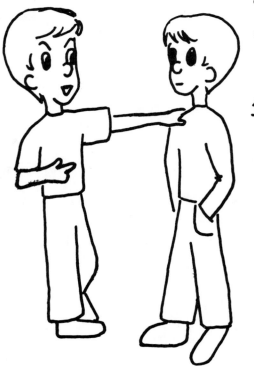

8. Your friend never invites you over to play.

9. You and your friend decide to go to the movies. You really want to see the movie in Theater 1, but your friend insists on seeing the movie in Theater 2.

10. You find out that someone you think is your friend is telling stories about you.

8 Growing Up for Girls

PURPOSE

The transition from latency to adolescence presents sexually abused girls and their caretakers with a new set of challenges. The physical changes that occur during this developmental stage awaken questions about sexual identity, body image, and dating. Some girls may wonder if they will ever begin menstruation or be able to become pregnant. In contrast, other girls reveal that they have always worried that they might become pregnant as a result of their molestation, even though it did not include sexual intercourse. Many girls are confused about what constitutes "purity" and may ask the therapists for clarification on the meaning of "being a virgin." Furthermore, caretakers' own discomfort with the sexual nature of their children's abuse and fears that their children may not be "normal" may contribute to the children's sense of having been damaged. This is compounded by the caretakers' lack of education or discomfort with sexuality, especially for those who have been victims of sexual abuse themselves.

Some girls react to the physical changes that occur during puberty with disgust and try to conceal their bodies with oversized or "boyish" clothing in an attempt to deny their sexuality. Others, whose counterphobic behavior gives them a false sense of mastery, may behave provocatively, thereby increasing their risk for further victimization. Regardless of the various manifestations of the sexual trauma, the girls' concept of growing up and their sexual identity are colored by frightening and confusing thoughts. They are prematurely exposed to inappropriate and involuntary sexual activity without enough knowledge or understanding about sex or the capacity to integrate the experience. This module provides an opportunity for the girls and their caretakers to learn about female sexual development, allaying myths and helping the girls to develop a more optimistic outlook about growing up and becoming women.

OBJECTIVES

1. Encourage the caretakers to pay attention to their children's sexualized behavior.
2. Normalize sexual curiosity in children.
3. Provide children and caretakers with accurate information about sexual development and reproduction.
4. Explore issues about sexual relationships.

5. Clarify the children's and caretakers' misconceptions about sexual abuse and future sexuality.
6. Permit caretakers to share their own feelings of disappointment about their daughters' "loss of innocence."

THERAPEUTIC CONSIDERATIONS

In order to increase the likelihood that girls and their caretakers will benefit from the information in this module, therapists must:

1. Be sensitive to the developmental differences that exist within the group. While some girls may still be prepubescent, others may have already reached puberty.
2. Recognize that levels of sexual knowledge and sophistication among group members may vary and that some girls may already be sexually active.
3. Respect caretakers' discomfort about discussing sex and sexuality with their children.
4. Understand the impact of cultural and religious beliefs on attitudes about sexual behavior.
5. Realize that normalizing sexual curiosity and behavior may increase awareness of guilt in some children, who found some aspects of the sexual molestation pleasurable.
6. Anticipate that the combination of male and female members in the caretakers' group may create some discomfort when sexuality is being discussed.
7. Clarify that while therapists facilitate the exploration of sexual identity issues, it is the caretakers' role to convey family values about sexuality.

ACTIVITIES FOR MODULE #8 (3 sessions)

1. A film about puberty

The children are shown one of the many excellent available films (see "Additional Resources" for one suggestion) that introduce sexual development at an age-appropriate level. This is a helpful tool in promoting a discussion about sexual development and allows the girls to begin to verbalize some of their fears about being "damaged" versus "normal." Following the film, children typically raise concerns about developing too early or too late in relation to other girls their age; confusion about male versus female sexual development; and questions about heterosexual relationships. Following the viewing of the film in one group, a girl took the opportunity to tell the others that she had just "started her period." In another group, a girl admitted frustration with her slow breast development compared with that of her friends.

In the caretakers' group, the adults:

a. View the same film that is selected for the children, and discuss their own confusion or ignorance about female sexual development. It is advisable to prepare the caretakers for this segment by allowing them to see the film well in advance of the children and to raise any concerns about what their girls may learn in group.

b. Consider what information in the film they think will be new to their children, and what information they think their children already know.

c. Express their concerns about "damage" to their children by the sexual abuse.

d. Explore what their own parents' attitudes were about sexuality and how this may have influenced their ability to talk with their children about sexual development and behavior.

2. Questions about sex

In this exercise, the girls are asked to anonymously write down on paper any questions they have about sex or puberty. This enables group members to ask questions without fears of feeling embarrassed or being teased. The therapists collect the questions and read them out loud. The group members are invited to respond if they think they know the answers, and the therapists offer clarifications and information. Some of the most common questions are, "How are babies made?", "Can you get pregnant without having sex?", "What is birth control?", "How old should a girl be before having sex?", "Will my boyfriend or husband be able to tell that I was molested?", "Am I still a virgin?", "How do people get AIDS?", and "What will boys think if they know I was molested?"

In the caretakers' group, the adults:

a. Discuss how they themselves learned about sex.

b. Consider how their children should learn about sex.

c. Examine how they react when their children ask them questions about sex and whether they allow discussion of sex in their homes.

d. Explore how they communicate their attitudes, values, and concerns about sex to their children.

3. When I Grow Up (Handout 8-1)

In this exercise, the therapists prepare a large poster board with pictures of women in a variety of adult roles, including various professional women (doctor, nurse, businesswoman, teacher), an athlete, a woman with a child, a model, various artists (dancer, musician), and a laborer. Each picture is designated with a number that the children can use when completing the handout. When numbers are used, the children can project their own ideas about the woman in each picture and are not limited by the labeling of the therapists. For example, the therapists might consider a picture of a woman with a child to be a "mother," while the girls might identify the picture as a "babysitter" or "therapist."

The children are shown the pictures and are asked to complete a handout that addresses their hopes and fears about becoming women and how their goals might be achieved. The therapists then use the answers to engage the girls in a discussion about their future and to focus on how each girl feels the molestation may affect her as an adult. For example, girls who feel "dirty" and "damaged" may see themselves as unworthy of becoming successful. This exercise explores common stereotypes about adult women and ways in which these interplay with sexual identity; it helps the girls begin to think about their images of themselves now and in the future. One girl selected the picture of the doctor because she wanted to be able to help children who had been molested. Another girl said she would "least like to be" the woman with the child because she never wanted to have sex.

In the caretakers' group, the adults:

a. Share their thoughts about what types of adults they think their daughters will become.

b. Predict which women on the collage their daughters will most likely identify with, and how these are similar or different from the roles they would wish for their daughters.

c. Compare their images of themselves as adults to their childhood fantasies of the types of adults they wanted to become.

d. Examine what childhood experiences influenced the images they have of themselves as adults.

e. Share concerns about their daughters' future.

ADDITIONAL RESOURCES

There are numerous excellent resources that present information about sexual development and behavior. These are some of the resources that have been found helpful.

1. Smallwood, S., & Walsh, S. (Producers). (1986). *What's happening to me? A guide to puberty* [Videotape]. Consolidated Productions.
2. Gitchel, S., & Foster, L. (1986). *Let's talk about . . . S-e-x.* (Available from Planned Parenthood of Central California, Fresno, CA)
3. Mayle, P. (1975). *What's happening to me?* Secaucus, NJ: Lyle Stuart.
4. Mayle, P. (1973). *Where did I come from?* Secaucus, NJ: Lyle Stuart.
5. Johnson, T. C. (1989). *Sexuality curriculum.* (Currently in progress at Children's Institute International, 711 South New Hampshire, Los Angeles, CA, 90005)

TREATMENT CHALLENGES

1. Some caretakers do not want to talk to their children about sex and may become angry or suspicious of the therapists for introducing sex education

in group. Therapists should acknowledge the caretakers' difficulty with this and reassure them that the purpose is not to teach the children more than they already know about sex, but to clarify misconceptions and provide accurate information. It may even be helpful to meet individually with a concerned caretaker. In the rare instances when caretakers continue to maintain that they do not want their children to be a part of this discussion, they can be given the option of not having their children attend group until this segment is completed. The authors are aware that excluding a child from any activity can lead to increased feelings of isolation and personal stigmatization and can alter the dynamics of the group as a whole. However, in all cases, therapists should respect the wishes of caretakers and not recapitulate feelings of victimization by insisting that children participate. This would most likely lead to premature withdrawal from the program, which is potentially more damaging and disruptive.

2. Therapists can anticipate high levels of anxiety among the children when sexual information is introduced. Therapists should normalize feelings of embarrassment and discomfort with the subject and encourage the girls to talk about the source of their anxiety (e.g., fear of learning that they are no longer "virgins," etc.).

3. Some children are intimidated by others who claim to know a lot about sex, and feel uncomfortable asking questions because they fear they may be ridiculed. Therapists should reassure the group that no one knows everything and that some people may think they have accurate information when in fact they do not. Children who are too shy to ask questions will have an opportunity to write them down or to ask the therapists in private.

Name: _____

When I Grow Up

1. How are these women alike? _____
_____

2. How are these women different? _____
_____

3. How do you think these various women feel? _____
_____

4. Which of these women would you most like to be when you grow up? _____
_____

Why? _____

5. What do you think your chances are of becoming this woman? _____
_____

6. What kinds of things would you have to do
to become this woman? _____
_____
_____

7. Which of these women would you least like
to be? _____
_____

Why? _____
_____

8. What has happened to you or what might happen
to you that could make you become like this
woman?
_____
_____
_____

MODULE 9 Growing Up for Boys

PURPOSE

The transition from latency to puberty in boys is often marked with confusion and reluctance to ask for clarification about the developing male body. For the male victim of sexual molestation, the emerging sexual identity and capacity to interact with peers is influenced by considerable shame, lack of self-esteem, and overwhelming fears about being considered "weak," "passive," or "gay." Boys are most often abused by offenders of the same sex, which incites cultural fears and myths about homosexuality. Male victims often believe they are fated to become homosexuals or that some "weakness" must have been perceived and exploited by the perpetrator. Boys frequently perceive homosexuality as a contagion they "catch" by virtue of a sexual experience with a male. The diminished sense of maleness can lead to extreme withdrawal from the peer group or aggressive overcompensation in an attempt to restore feelings of being intact, and gives the illusion of a restored masculinity.

Caretakers also fear damage to boys' masculinity and struggle in their effort to understand and contain their children's acting-out behavior. The adults perpetuate and reinforce these beliefs due to their own discomfort which at times takes the form of blaming their children for having "allowed" the molestation to occur. Boys and caretakers share in the societal expectation that males should be in control and strong, which is inconsistent with the idea of males' being sexually victimized. It is often difficult for boys to separate their own image of themselves from their caretakers' hysteria and condemnations of gay men. Furthermore, adults who have some emotional attachment to the perpetrators frequently seek to alleviate their own anxiety by telling the boys that the perpetrators were similarly abused as children. As a result, boys often fear that they too will be unable to control such behavior.

This module attempts to provide appropriate information about the normal changes signaling advancing sexuality, and to uncover and dispel myths about the damaging effects of the sexual abuse. The male therapists attempt to create an arena where appropriate masculine identifications are reinforced and abusive or aggressive behavior is discouraged.

OBJECTIVES

1. Clarify misperceptions about the relationship of sexual molestation to homosexuality.

151

2. Reduce shame over feelings of helplessness related to the molestation.

3. Provide appropriate information about sexual development to normalize confusing sexual feelings.

4. Emphasize the positive attributes of group members and male therapists as a means of providing options for male identifications, thereby reducing inappropriate attempts to establish masculinity.

5. Address group members' concerns about entering male–female relationships.

6. Encourage caretakers to discuss issues of sexuality with their children more openly.

7. Explore caretakers' anger at male children for "having allowed" the abuse to occur.

THERAPEUTIC CONSIDERATIONS

In order to increase the likelihood that boys and their caretakers will benefit from the information in this module, therapists must:

1. Be sensitive to the developmental differences of group members that are relevant to the presentation of sex education.

2. Clarify that while therapists facilitate the exploration of sexual identity issues, it is the caretakers' role to convey family values about sexuality.

3. Recognize that normalization of sexual feelings and responses may raise group members' anxiety about feelings of arousal experienced during their molestation.

4. Expect that any discussion of feelings of helplessness that contradict male role expectations will require therapeutic intervention to empower boys to act assertively rather than aggressively. Therapists should be prepared to assimilate previous material from Module #7 when applicable.

5. Communicate comfort with sex education material to help diminish the expected anxieties of children and caretakers.

6. Accept that therapists are inevitably limited in their ability to penetrate ingrained and culturally reinforced stereotypes and myths about acceptable male behavior.

7. Recognize that boys who are sexually abused by women may have the additional conflict of feeling victimized, yet viewing the molestation as a sexual conquest.

8. Expect that as some group members explore male identifications, unresolved feelings about their impoverished relationships with their own fathers will emerge.

ACTIVITIES FOR MODULE #9 (3 sessions)

1. A Film about Sexual Development

In this exercise, the boys are shown a film (see "Additional Resources" for one suggestion) about puberty and reproduction. This film should describe actual physical changes in appearance, the physiology of sexual arousal and orgasm, and the development of the capacity to reproduce. Therapists then facilitate a discussion focusing on questions that group members have about puberty, emphasizing it as a normal stage of development. Frequently this material raises issues related to the sexual abuse, and therapists should keep in mind the dynamics of male abuse victims to guide their interventions during this module. One boy, after learning that erections can occur as a result of a wide variety of sexual and nonsexual stimuli, was able to reveal his shame over having an erection during his molestation. Another group member was able to admit that he acted as if he knew everything about sex so that no one would think that he was a "sissy." The therapists were able to connect these disclosures with the fear of being damaged.

In the caretakers' group:

a. The adults view the same film before their children do, and discuss their own confusion or lack of understanding of male sexual development.
b. The caretakers explore their discomfort about discussing sexuality with their children and develop strategies to allow for more open communications.
c. The adults are encouraged to share their concerns regarding the effect of each boy's molestation on the course of his sexual development. At this point, caretakers often begin to verbalize their fears that the boys may become homosexual or eventually victimize others.

2. Questions about Sex

Following the discussion about the film in the preceding exercise, the group members are asked to anonymously write down at least one additional question they have about sex. The boys are told that these questions will be discussed between the therapists and answered the following week. The confidentiality of the questioner and lack of specific focus in the instructions allow areas of special concern or conflict for each group member to surface. During this exercise, these questions are read aloud and discussed. Some of the most common questions are: "If sex feels so good, why don't people do it all of the time?", "Do people have to have sex when they grow up?", "Why are some guys gay?", "Why do some people have sex with children?", and "Are all molesters 'fags'?" These questions allow the therapists to address a variety of concerns, such as conflict over pleasurable feelings experienced during the molestation; wishes to avoid normal sexual development and intimacy; fears of having been somehow transformed into homosexuals; and disguised concerns about their own capacity to perpetrate. This is often the time when boys begin to verbalize concerns about being or becoming gay, and some group members may admit to having molested a peer or younger child. This activity allows therapists to help the children explore and validate their feelings about these very charged issues. However, dealing directly with the topics of homosexuality or sexual perpetration often poses a threat to the fragile defensive structure of these latency-age children. Therefore, these issues should not be pursued unless there are group members who are open to talking about them.

In the caretakers' group, the adults:

a. Engage in the same exercise, increasing their empathy for the anxiety that their children experience in regard to sexuality.

b. Explore the importance of open communication about sexual issues to eliminate the misperceptions that can develop in an atmosphere of secrecy and stigmatization.

3. When I Grow Up (Handout 9-1)

In this exercise, the therapists prepare a large poster board with pictures of men in a variety of adult roles, including several professional men (doctor, businessman in a suit, teacher), several athletes (football player, baseball player, surfer), a man with a child, various artists (dancer, musician), a laborer, a daredevil, a soldier, and a policeman. Each picture is designated with a number that the children can use when completing the handout. When numbers are used, the children can project their own ideas about the man in each picture and are not limited by the labeling of the therapists. For example, the therapists might consider a picture of a man balanced on a beam to be a "construction worker," while the boys might identify the man as a "daredevil."

The boys are shown the pictures and are asked to complete a handout which addresses their hopes and fears about becoming men and considers how goals might be achieved. The therapists then use the answers to engage the boys in a discussion about their future and to focus on how each boy feels the molestation may affect him as an adult. One boy praised the strength and weapons of the soldier as able to insure that no one could hurt him, while at the same time identifying the soldier as always being scared and therefore needing a threatening facade.

In the caretakers' group, the adults:

a. Participate in the same exercise to examine their own expectations regarding adult male roles.

b. Explore the conflict and sense of failure that they and their children experience in attempting to integrate the commonly held expectation that men should be able to avoid victimization with the reality of the abuse experience.

c. Help caretakers to reinforce flexible and appropriate male identifications, ones that promote openness and assertiveness.

ADDITIONAL RESOURCES

Again, there are numerous excellent resources that present information about sexual development and behavior. The resources listed in Module #8 for girls can also be used with boys. In addition, the authors have found the following videotape helpful:

1. Franco, D., & Shepard, D. (Producers). (1979). *Am I normal? A film about male puberty* [Videotape]. Boston: Boston Family Planning Project.

TREATMENT CHALLENGES

1. Some caretakers may be unwilling to have their children learn about sexual development, either due to their own discomfort with sexuality or for fear that their children will be overstimulated. Therapists should attempt to understand the adults' concerns and clarify the purpose of presenting the material. If the caretakers remain firm in their resistance, then the children may be excused from that group session. As discussed in Module #8, therapists must consider the alternatives: the consequences of exclusion from the activity, and the risk that insistence may lead to early termination by a family.

2. For those children who continue to feel damaged, the need to behave aggressively or portray themselves as unaffected may become more pronounced. Therapists must be aware that these defenses are necessary and may best be explored in individual treatment without the added pressure of peers whom a boy wishes to impress.

3. During the discussion of sexual development, some boys may ridicule other group members for asking questions. Children often berate others for not knowing about sex, regardless of the degree of their own knowledge. The therapists should not demand that a provoking child know the answers, but rather should focus on reinforcing the courage of the child who makes himself vulnerable enough to pose the questions.

Name: _____

When I Grow Up

1. How are these men alike? _____
   _____
   _____

2. How are these men different? _____
   _____
   _____

3. How do you think these various men feel? _____
   _____
   _____

4. Which of these men would you most like to be when
   you grow up? _____
   Why? _____

5. What do you think your chances are of becoming this man? _____
   _____

6. What kinds of things would you have to do to become this man? _____
   _____

7. Which of these men would you least like to be? _____
   _____ Why? _____
   _____

8. What has happened to you or what might happen to you that could make you
   become like this man? _____
   _____

MODULE 10 Saying Good-Bye

PURPOSE

The conclusion of group is often experienced by children and their caretakers with marked ambivalence. Although there are feelings of accomplishment about fulfilling their commitment to the group treatment, and expressions of relief as they are eager to "get on with their lives," the children and the adults begin to mourn an anticipated loss. These groups foster strong supportive relationships because of the sharing of very personal and painful experiences. Group members who were once isolated and silent have found a safe place, and there is sadness about leaving the structure which group provides and saying good-bye to special friends. One mother expressed the wish that she "be weaned slowly" at the end, because group was the "only" place where she could really talk about her experience.

Imposed termination not only evokes memories of past losses and rejections, but reactivates feelings of helplessness. Termination may occur before everyone feels ready to end and before individual goals are reached. However, latency-age children rarely verbalize difficulties with termination. Instead, the therapists must anticipate and look for denial, regression, increased aggression or withdrawal, and devaluing of the group and the therapists as evidence of the reaction to and the defense against loss and feelings of abandonment. Group members must be helped to acknowledge that the group work is completed. The way in which the group experience is brought to a close will influence the degree to which gains are maintained. This module focuses exclusively on the special issues of termination—allowing the children and the caretakers to formally end group treatment and providing closure to a long-term intense experience.

OBJECTIVES

1. Encourage the exploration of feelings about termination in relation to past rejection and loss.
2. Permit positive feelings about completing the group program, and reinforce readiness to end group treatment.
3. Facilitate a review of the group process, focusing on meaningful group experiences as well as acknowledgement of personal gains.
4. Determine the need for future intervention for each group participant, and provide feedback and recommendations to the families.

THERAPEUTIC CONSIDERATIONS

In order to help group members and group leaders to have a positive termination experience, therapists must:

1. Acknowledge that there are always additional gains to be made by keeping the group together.
2. Understand that the inevitable regression that occurs as a response to termination is an attempt to cope with ending and is not necessarily indicative of a need for future treatment.
3. Predict that caretakers can expect some exacerbation of their children's difficulties or a reappearance of symptoms around the time of termination.
4. Accept the limitations of the group treatment program, recognizing that outside events occurring in the life of each child may have a more profound effect on that child's behavior and emotional development.
5. Recognize that some children may continue to suffer from severe symptomatology in spite of their experience in group.
6. Appreciate the importance of the therapists' revealing their sense of loss as well.
7. Acknowledge that while some children and their caretakers will benefit from additional individual/family treatment, there may not be sufficient staff time available to provide these services. Furthermore, some families will not follow through with recommendations for continued intervention.

ACTIVITIES FOR MODULE #10 (4 sessions)

1. Since I've Been in Group (Handout 10-1)

In this activity, the children complete a checklist covering some feelings and behaviors that may have changed during the course of group treatment. The therapists use the responses and their own observations to provide objective feedback and evaluate individual progress and development. In one group, a girl marked "a lot" to the statement, "I can talk to my parents." She had been silent for 4 years before disclosing molestation by her father, but was able to inform her mother immediately when a neighbor exposed himself. This girl attributed her improved self-protectiveness to validation she received in the group, which decreased her feelings of helplessness. Therapists can also use the responses to this handout to assess the need for further intervention. One child marked "not at all" to the statement, "The people in my family get along together." This alerted the therapists that unresolved conflict in the home might require additional family treatment.

In the caretakers' group, the adults consider:

a. The changes they have witnessed in their children over the course of the group.

b. The changes they have experienced in themselves as a result of participation in group treatment.

c. Possible disappointment when their children continue to demonstrate serious problem behavior.

2. My Group (Handout 10-2)

In this exercise, the children are asked to complete a handout that identifies possible feelings about termination and asks the children to evaluate their group treatment experience. The therapists engage the children in a general discussion about the ending of group. The group members are encouraged to share what they found most helpful about group, as well as aspects of the treatment they would change if they were planning the next group. Children usually express positive feelings about group, stating that it was "fun" and often focusing on the opportunity to make new friends and to learn that other children have had similar experiences. There are also many group members who would prefer "more snacks or playtime" and "less talking."

In the caretakers' group, the adults:

a. Consider how their children feel about termination.

b. Share their own reactions to the end of group treatment.

c. Address the most helpful aspects of the group experience for themselves and their children.

d. Provide feedback to the therapists about the treatment program by completing the "Group Evaluation Form" (Handout 10-3).

3. Saying Good-Bye (Handout 10-4)

In this activity, the children use a structured letter to say good-bye to each group member and each therapist. The therapists also write a letter to each child, providing positive feedback about group participation and progress. Once the letters are completed, the children are each given all of their letters, which they read aloud in the group. This is always a very positive experience when children learn that they are valued and will be missed. Some children may also wish to write good-bye letters to group members who terminated prematurely. Therapists should encourage this effort to gain closure, agreeing to make certain that the letters are mailed.

In the caretakers' group, the adults:

a. Participate in the same exercise as the children and have the opportunity to reinforce each other's contribution to the group experience.

4. Good-Bye Party

The final session should be reserved for a farewell party, and the therapists can encourage the children to plan the activities and refreshments. At the end of the party, the children are given their folders with all of the materials they have used throughout the group. Therapists may also want to give each child an inexpensive age-appropriate gift. The caretakers are also encouraged to plan their own party, and therapists can consider combining the two groups for the last part of this final celebration.

TREATMENT CHALLENGES

1. Many caretakers have difficulty crediting the treatment with positive changes they observe in their children. One mother believed that her daughter had become more assertive because she was now older. Therapists should not try to defend the value of group treatment, but should focus on how the caretakers have contributed to their children's progress.

2. Once termination is announced, some caretakers will want to end early or begin missing sessions. One father did not attend the second-to-last group meeting because he had an opportunity to play golf. Other caretakers directly devalue the importance of formal termination, questioning the need for a party at the last meeting. It is usually helpful to predict these reactions. The therapists should explore feelings about ending treatment in the context of past losses, and reinforce the importance of allowing the children and adults to celebrate their accomplishment.

3. Some caretakers fear that their children need further group treatment and want guarantees about future adjustment. "Will my child be OK?" is often asked. While reinforcing the benefits of a group therapy experience, therapists must always discuss a child's capacity to "survive" sexual molestation in the context of prior ego strengths, external life circumstances, support of significant adults, and anticipated regression points that correspond to developmental milestones. Therapists should encourage the adults to consider the growth they have observed in their children. Caretakers should also be reassured that each child's progress will be evaluated to determine further treatment needs.

4. Some children become concerned that the therapists are recommending more treatment for them when other children are being discharged from the program. Therapists must first address such a child's concerns about the "meaning" of additional treatment. Attempts should then be made to enlist the caretakers in clarifying for the child that continued intervention is not a sign of the child's failure, but the family's decision to continue working on issues that are still affecting the child's life.

Other children may insist that in spite of therapists' plans for termination, they still need further intervention. One girl expressed dismay that she was the only group member who would be discharged completely from the program, having no further contact with the therapists. In some cases, therapists may arrange to meet with families on an intermittent basis, with the explicit understanding that this will lead to eventual termination.

Name: _____

Since I've been in group:

	a lot	some	a little	not at all
1. I can talk about what happened to me.	—	—	—	—
2. I tell people what I need.	—	—	—	—
3. Other kids like to be with me.	—	—	—	—
4. I feel safer.	—	—	—	—
5. I have good things to say.	—	—	—	—
6. People understand how I feel.	—	—	—	—
7. I can talk to my parents.	—	—	—	—
8. I am happy at school.	—	—	—	—
9. I can tell people when I am angry.	—	—	—	—
10. The people in my family get along together.	—	—	—	—

Name: _____

My Group

1. I feel _____ that group is coming to an end.

2. The hardest thing about group was _____
   _____.

3. I wish that _____.

4. Being a part of this group has been _____
   _____ for me.

5. I wish that _____.

6. Part of me is _____ that group is over, but I also
   feel _____.

7. It was _____ making new friends.

8. I felt _____ and _____ telling what
   happened to me.

9. If I were running the group, I would have more _____
   _____ and less _____.

10. These are some things I want to say to the group: _____
    _____
    _____
    _____.

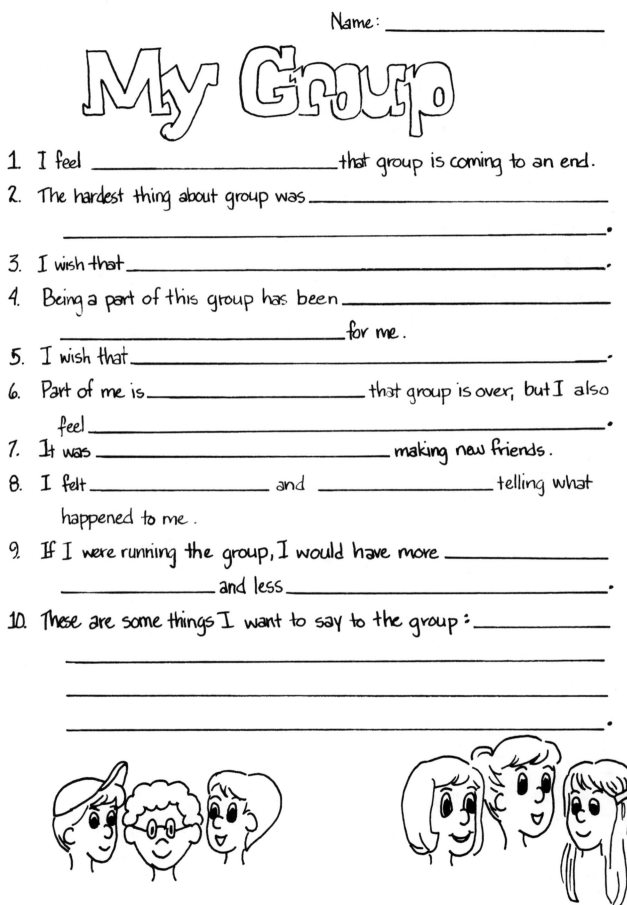

HANDOUT 10-3: PARENT EVALUATION OF GROUP

		A lot	Some what	A little	Not at all
1.	The therapists were clear in the preparing me for the issues my child would be discussing.	___	___	___	___
2.	The therapists were clear in preparing me for the issues I would be discussing.	___	___	___	___
3.	My feelings about group have changed.	___	___	___	___

How?_____

_____

		A lot	Some what	A little	Not at all
4.	I understand the importance of my participation in my child's treatment.	___	___	___	___
5.	I feel that I better understand my child. How?	___	___	___	___

_____

| 6. | I have seen positive changes in my child. | | | | |

Please describe._____   ___ ___ ___ ___

_____

| 7. | I have seen positive changes in myself. | | | | |

Please describe._____   ___ ___ ___ ___

_____

8. What about group has been most helpful to you?_____

_____

_____

9. What about group has been most helpful to your child?_____

_____

_____

10. If you were the group therapist, what might you do differently?_____

_____

_____

Date: _____

Goodbye Letter

Dear_____,

　　We have known each other now for a long time.

When I first met you _____

_____

but after I got to know you better I _____

_____.

Having you in group has _____

_____and I will miss

_____.

I'm glad you were in group because _____

_____,

and I want to thank you _____

_____.

　I hope that_____

_____

_____.

_____

_____

P.S. _____

_____